Dairy-free & / or

Wheat-free & / or

Soya-free BUT

Always Totally Nut-free

Family Cookbook

Clare Constant
Suzanne Wood

www.allergyfamilycookbook.com

Strategic Business Transformation Ltd

Published by Strategic Business Transformation Ltd.
Anstey Park House, Anstey Road Alton, Hampshire, GU34 2RL
First published 2007
Second Edition 2008

While the authors of this book have made every effort to ensure that the information contained in this book is as accurate and up-to-date as possible at the time of publication, medical and pharmaceutical knowledge is constantly changing and the application of it to particular circumstances depends on many factors. Therefore it is recommended that readers always consult a qualified medical specialist for individual advice. This book should not be used as an alternative to seeking specialist medical advice which should be sought before any action is taken. The authors and publisher cannot be held responsible for any errors and omissions that may be found in the text, or any actions that may be taken by a reader as a result of any reliance on or use of the information contained in the text which is taken entirely at the reader's own risk. The authors do not endorse, approve or assume responsibility for any product, brand or company. Within the text the presence (or absence) of a product does not constitute approval (or disapproval) by the authors.

The authors would particularly like to thank Dr Diab Haddad of St Peter's Hospital, Chertsey, Honorary Consultant in Paediatric Allergy at the Evelina Children's Hospital, St Thomas' London for his invaluable help in the reading and checking of the manuscript.
Clare Constant would like to dedicate this book with love to: DG and to Matthew, Madeleine and Sophie Constant, Raymond and Margaret Morgan, Michael and Janet Morgan, Dominic Morgan and Tony Wiltshire.
Suzanne Wood would like to thank Phil, Melanie and Andrew for tasting all the recipes and giving their honest opinions. Each recipe had to meet with their hard-won approval before it was allowed in the book. Thanks are also due to parents Margaret and Peter, and in-laws Audrey and Martin, as well as Phil Drake – our eagle-eyed recipe proof-reader. We would also like to thank Peter Carrow of Carrow Design for the brilliant cover (www.carrowdesign.com).

FOREWORD

With the increasing awareness of allergies as a relatively common cause of ill health, the number of people, particularly children, who are following some sort of food avoidance, has dramatically increased. As many parents will know, it is difficult, at the best of times, to get children to consume an adequate diet that will meet their nutritional needs. To attempt to achieve this, while still having to follow the various restrictions which are frequently imposed on the diets of children with food allergies, can become an impossible task.

There is thus a real need for easy to follow, quick solutions to help families cater for the needs of allergic individuals yet maintain the nutritional value and taste of prepared foods. If such dishes could also tempt other members of the family then one meal can be prepared for the whole family and the sense of normality and family experience would not be undermined. This book offers recipes which help to meet these needs and address these issues.

Drawing on their own personal and family experiences, the authors offer very practical, ingenious and creative solutions for the preparation of nutritious, healthy and tasty meals, while still staying away from the various types of foods that allergic members of the family should avoid.

As is repeatedly stated within this work, it is wrong to jump to conclusions and the diagnosis of food allergy should only be made by qualified health professionals such as a GP or a Paediatrician. Imposing food restrictions unnecessarily serves no good purpose and can lead to harm. Once the diagnosis of an allergy is made and the recommendation to restrict various types of food in the diet has been given by dieticians and qualified health professionals, this book will make the task much easier and will provide solutions for the whole family. This is done in a way which should make preparing food, once again, an enjoyable uncomplicated task, filled with lots of fun.

Dr Diab F Haddad MD MRCPCH, Consultant Paediatrician St Peter's Hospital, Chertsey, Honorary Consultant in Paediatric Allergy at the Evelina Children's Hospital, St Thomas' London

Content

Useful information:

Recipes:

Indexes:

1: What is food intolerance?

The term food intolerance is used to mean the inability to tolerate certain foods either due to allergy or other causes. When the sufferer comes into contact with that food then the body reacts adversely and produces symptoms. **Food intolerance** may result from a wide range of different causes such as the body failing to produce a particular enzyme needed to digest the food, or having an immune reaction against the food which is referred to as allergy. Therefore, **food allergy** is one particular form of food intolerance. If someone has a food allergy it is because the immune system in their body reacts to the food causing adverse effects. A common mechanism in which the body reacts is by producing antibodies to the food - frequently of the IgE (immunoglobulin E) class.

An important part of the body's immune system is its **mast cells** which are mostly found in the skin, soft tissue, organs and joints. They work by producing chemicals such as **histamine**. As the mast cells do their work, sufferers experience unpleasant symptoms such as swelling, inflammation and excessive mucous production in the regions where the mast cells' chemicals act.

Antihistamines help the allergic symptoms to fade. This is why doctors may prescribe an antihistamine medicine for allergy sufferers to take in order to reduce the effect of symptoms when they experience an allergic reaction.

The speed at which individual's bodies respond to a food to which they are allergic can vary enormously. In extreme cases the sufferer may react violently within a few seconds and experience the life-threatening symptoms of **anaphylactic reaction**. For others, their symptoms may occur days after the food was ingested, making the process of pinpointing which food is causing the problem much more difficult.

Complete avoidance of the problem food will ensure that allergic symptoms caused by it are no longer triggered. In extreme cases this may mean ensuring that there is no possibility of the sufferer inhaling or coming into contact with even minute traces of the problem food.

Diseases caused by foods

Coeliac disease is an autoimmune disease triggered by gluten, a protein found in wheat, barley and rye. It is estimated that 1 in 100 people have Coeliac disease. (Bingley PJ et al, 2004) Longitudinal studies of parents and children study team. *British Medical Journal.* 328, 322-3; West, J. et al (2003) Seroprevalence, correlates, and characteristics of undetected coeliac disease in England. *Gut;* 52:960–965.)

In Coeliac disease it is the gluten (which occurs in wheat, barley and rye) which causes the body to produce antibodies that attack its own tissues. Tiny finger like projections, called villi, become damaged and flattened, leading to a reduced surface area for absorbing nutrients. As a result people with undiagnosed Coeliac disease can experience nutritional deficiency.

Dermatitis Herpetiformis is also caused by inability to digest wheat. Once again, the only cure is to eliminate wheat from the diet.

Although there has been discussion in the media about possible links between gluten, dairy and soya with other diseases there is still a lot of research to be carried out in this area.

Allergic reaction *(IgE mediated type)*

How fast is the reaction?	What is the body doing?	Can the body ever react differently?
Can be rapid – within a minute or up to two hours later.	IgE antibodies in the immune system can react to a minute amount of the problem food. The histamine reaction is rapid and violent with the result that its effects can be life-threatening e.g. anaphylactic reaction.	The cells producing IgE antibodies have a memory. Doctors generally expect most children who are allergic to cow's milk to outgrow the allergy by the time they are five. However, allergies to nuts and fish tend to be permanent. In this case lifelong avoidance of the problem food is the only solution.

Intolerance

How fast is the reaction?	What is the body doing?	Can the body ever react differently?
Can be rapid or much slower depending on the cause – symptoms may appear after several hours or even days later.	The body is unable to tolerate a food for some reason e.g. it does not produce the enzyme needed to digest it, or the immune system treats the food as an enemy invader and releases antibodies in an allergic reaction.	This depends on the cause of the intolerance. If, for example, the body does not produce an enzyme such as lactase (needed to digest the lactose in milk) then the sufferer will remain intolerant. In other situations intolerance may only be a temporary situation.

2: Identifying a child's food sensitivity

Most of the time food is something we enjoy and, for a child, eating is a particularly important part of life. From babyhood, eating can provide happy and stimulating experiences through the introduction of new foods, and the social interaction that accompanies mealtimes. Alternatively, struggling to eat a food we dislike, or experiencing a stressful mealtime, can create an unhappy memory that we carry for the whole of our lives.

Increasingly, however, children's reaction to food has nothing to do with its novelty, its texture, the behaviour of others while they are eating, or the memories associated with a particular food. Instead certain food constituents cause the child's body to react in an unpleasant, or even alarming, way.

If the reaction is a more dramatic collapse, such as in anaphylactic reaction, you may be in no doubt as to the cause. But, sometimes, symptoms from eating a problem food are a lot subtler. Is ongoing stomach-ache and diarrhoea the result of a long-lasting infection, or is her body reacting badly to a particular food? Is he hyperactive, or are certain foods triggering his difficult behaviour? Is this endless fuss about 'tummy ache' after breakfast caused by anxiety about school, or is the milk on her cereal making her feel unwell?

So how can you tell if a food is making your child ill?

Symptoms that may suggest an allergy or food intolerance

Skin problems

rashes – particularly itchy lesions and hives
dry flaky skin
psoriasis

Digestion problems

In babies:
colic
vomiting
poor appetite and failure to grow
rancid smelling faeces
diarrhoea or constipation

In older children and adults:
frequent mouth ulcers
catarrh
persistent coughing
an uncomfortable bloated feeling in the abdomen
stomach pains
gut cramps
vomiting
flatulence
diarrhoea
constipation

Whole body symptoms

anaphylactic reaction
flu-like aches and pains in joints and muscles
sinus problems
sneezing, and constant runny nose
headaches or migraine
lethargy
loss of concentration

Mental and emotional symptoms

Some nutrition experts believe that sometimes the following symptoms may also be linked to food intolerance but this is currently unproven:

anxiety panic attacks
Attention Deficit Hyperactive Disorder (ADHD)
chronic fatigue
depression
hyperactivity (and bedwetting) in children
migraines
strong food cravings
sleep disorders

Warning!

Many of the symptoms in the lists above can also be signs that your child has a different underlying illness! Take him or her to the doctor to discuss your concerns <u>before</u> making any changes to your child's diet.

Investigating the symptoms

Since the more severe allergic reactions happen so quickly the diagnosis is usually obvious. However, if your child experiences a number of the milder symptoms listed earlier, it may be necessary to keep a food diary (see p13-16) to help your doctor to work out whether there is a link with any particular food.

It is important to note that many of the symptoms listed can also be indicators that your child is suffering from a different illness, or disease. This is why it is *essential* to work with your doctor, health visitor, or dietician to determine the real cause of your child's ill health and what steps you should take to improve it, rather than going it alone. Even if you feel sure that a particular food is causing the problem, you need to act with the help of a health professional. Stopping your child from eating a food that usually forms a significant part of their diet without replacing the missing nutrients could leave them with the far greater long-term problems of malnutrition, vitamin or mineral deficiency.

Case study
Jack was bottle-fed from 6 months but every day his mother, Rachel, struggled to get him to feed: 'By the time he was crawling, I used to chase him round the room with a bottle, forcing him to drink it.' To make things worse, Jack didn't gain weight, was constantly miserable, and his stools smelt rancid – like curdled fat.

These symptoms helped the paediatrician to diagnose milk allergy. Once a nutritionally balanced, dairy-free milk alternative was prescribed, and Rachel eliminated all cow's milk from his diet, Jack began to thrive. 'Now I can't feed him fast enough,' Rachel laughs.

Keeping a food diary

Writing down everything your child eats or drinks for 14 days and how they felt after each meal or snack is a first step to working out whether he may have a food allergy or intolerance. You can show the diary to your child's doctor or dietician to help them to make a diagnosis and advise you about the best way to improve your child's diet. The other advantage of a food diary is that it can also help you to work out whether your child is eating a healthy, balanced diet.

You need to keep the diary for two weeks so that there is enough evidence of any patterns. It can be set out like the one on the following pages. Start by writing down everything your child eats and drinks and at what time of day. Keep a record of their symptoms and what time they appear. An older child could make their own notes but you may have to promise not to nag if they are going to be able to admit to chips and chocolate bars every day for lunch! Explaining the purpose of keeping the food diary and the potential benefit of keeping it should encourage them to co-operate, especially as you are empowering them with a tool that can help them to find a way to feel better.

Once the diary is completed, pinpoint the times your child was most ill, and work out a list of ingredients in the foods eaten in the past day or two. In the food diary on the following pages, the dinner on Tuesday that made Jasmine vomit included two common problem foods: wheat and milk. In fact her dinner was loaded with dairy products because macaroni cheese contains cheese, milk and butter or margarine, and there was more cheese and butter or margarine in the cheesecake, which she had with cream.

Next, check the other times your child felt unwell and see if these are related to the intake of the same ingredients. Finally, look at the times when your child felt better and ask yourself: had she avoided the problem ingredients for a while before this period of no problem symptoms.

Jasmine's food diary suggests that she is reacting to milk because she feels unwell most of the day on Monday when she has a milky breakfast, cheese and chocolate for lunch, chocolate and butter in her afternoon snack, and milk in her custard at tea-time. She feels much healthier after breakfast and lunch on Tuesday – until she has her dairy-laden dinner.

Even with a food diary you may still find it difficult to be absolutely sure that you have correctly identified the cause of your child's allergy or intolerance correctly. This is why it is so important to share your suspicions with your child's doctor or dietician who can arrange for your child to be tested before making any long-term dietary changes.

Jasmine's Food Diary

Week 1 Monday

Meal	Time	Food	Symptoms
breakfast	7.45am	rice pops + milk milky hot chocolate	stomach ache before going to school
snack	10.30am	apple + water	stomach ache has eased but very lethargic
lunch	12.30pm	cheese sandwich, grapes, orange juice drink chocolate biscuit	stomach ache and sniffing a lot
snack	4.00pm	chocolate cake	headache
dinner	6.00pm	Spaghetti Bolognese, apple pie and orange squash	feeling a bit better in the evening, sniffing less

Week 1 Tuesday

Meal	Time	Food	Symptoms
breakfast	8.00am	Toast + dairy free margarine + honey + orange juice	felt 'fine', no sign of a cold
break	10.30am	apple + water	
lunch	12.30pm	tuna sandwich crisps apple juice cereal bar	
snack	4.00pm	cola drink	
dinner	6.00pm	macaroni cheese, cheese cake + cream + cup of tea with milk	vomited half an hour after dinner + 'cold' symptoms returned for rest of evening

Summary

- If your child is reacting to a particular food you will be able to spot unpleasant physical (and sometimes mental) symptoms after they eat it.

- In the case of a food allergy of the immediate type, identifying the problem food is usually fairly straightforward. With delayed forms of allergy or intolerance it can be much harder. Keeping a food diary can help.

- Ask your health professional to confirm whether food intolerance or allergy (rather than any underlying illness) is the cause of your child's problem.

- Once the diagnosis of allergy or intolerance is made, removing the problem food from your child's diet and replacing the missing nutrients should restore your child's health.

- The new diet should contain lots of fresh vegetables, fruit and protein.

- Using the recipes in this book will ensure that you can provide a variety of healthy, interesting meals

3: A Healthy Restricted Diet?

Changing information in the media about which foods are healthy and which are unhealthy can make us confused about what to feed our family.

Even once you think you know what to give them, putting it into practice may be a different matter. Children can be very fussy about what they will or won't put in their mouths. If you have to combine this with the stress of racing round a supermarket after work, it is all too easy to end up serving lots of highly processed foods midweek before sinking into junk food hell at weekends.

Add to this a new need to restrict a member of your family's diet because of an allergy or intolerance and you could easily feel on stress overload. In reality though, a healthy diet is the same for everyone: it is one that meets the needs of the body, helping it to work effectively and efficiently. To remain healthy each of us needs to have: water, protein, carbohydrate, fat, fibre, vitamins and minerals.

In 2005 the UK Government published seven tips for eating healthily telling you that you are doing well if, every day, you can persuade each member of your family to eat:

- Meals based on starchy foods
- Eat lots of fruit and vegetables
- Eat more fish
- Cut down on saturated fat and sugar
- Try to eat no more than 6g of salt a day (no salt should be added to food for toddlers and babies)
- Drink plenty of water
- Do not skip breakfast

Most people know they should eat <u>at least</u> 5 portions of fruit or vegetables and that the majority should be vegetables, but did you know it's a good idea to try and eat a variety of different colours? (E.g. red tomato, orange carrots, green broccoli, yellow pepper, apple etc.) If you are not sure about what proportion of different foods your family should eat then take a look at the eatwell plate which you can view at www.food.gov.uk.

Since children can only take in smaller quantities of food and yet are growing so rapidly, a child aged under two needs to eat more nutrient and energy-dense foods. It is important to ensure that the diet of all children is rich in iron and calcium.

To this end, make sure that the fruit and vegetables are fresh or frozen; and that the food is mostly unprocessed. The best way to ensure that each member of the family has enough mineral and vitamin-rich fruit and vegetables is to find ways to include them at every meal. Apart from the obvious plate of 'meat and two veg', try including:

- fruit juice or fruit smoothies at breakfast or as part of their packed lunch;
- fresh or dried fruit as snacks;
- vegetable sticks to eat dips;
- adding hidden vegetables and fruit in pasta and curry sauces, salads and cakes;
- fruit-based puddings.

The recipes in this book will help you to find ways to encourage even the fussiest eater to consume their 5+ portions every day.

If a very young child is unable to eat dairy products then making sure that she has enough protein, and eats enough calorie-rich foods to gain weight, can seem quite daunting.

A dietician may recommend two meat meals a day, and that high quantities of calorie-rich fat and sugar are included in the child's diet. This can be achieved through adding dairy-free margarine to vegetables, frying foods, and eating more cakes and biscuits.

Understandably this may go against your adult notions of healthy eating and you may be worried about the long-term effects on a child's health. However, it is vital to follow the dietician's advice.

You can try positively to influence all your children's future health by ensuring that they consume a rich variety of fruits and vegetables loaded with antioxidants such as broccoli, carrots, sweet potato, etc.

Bear in mind, also, that as they grow older children may develop a more mature digestive system so that in the future their diet can be reviewed and re-balanced.

Change the recipes as your children grow

Babies and toddlers who are very allergic to a number of different foods are often put on a very restricted diet to prevent them from developing further problems before their digestive and immune systems have matured. The list of banned foods is likely to include these common allergens: cow's milk, soya, egg, wheat, fish and nuts.

As the child grows older, the dietician will suggest which of these foods to try re-introducing into your child's diet. However, if your child's allergic reactions have been very strong, they may arrange for them to spend a day in hospital while being challenged with a particular food under medical supervision. Once the child is over three years old, then skin prick tests and the RAST blood tests will be carried out. These are useful in helping the paediatrician to diagnose an allergic reaction.

In this book, the recipes in the baby section do not include any of these six allergens listed above. In the toddler recipe section they are still avoided with the exception of two cake recipes where a small proportion of egg is included. (This is because cooked egg in a biscuit or cake is one of the first foods your child will be encouraged to try). While your child must avoid all egg, try using egg replacer in recipes. Egg replacer is sold in supermarkets or you can make it yourself: 1 egg = 1tbsp potato flour + 2tbsp water + ¼ tsp xanthan gum.

By the time they reach school age most children grow out of their reactions to the small quantities of cooked egg included in some recipes. For this reason the later recipe sections include egg. Although the good news is that the majority of children outgrow their reaction to cow's milk and soya by the age of five, the recipes in this book were developed with those who are not so fortunate in mind. Therefore dairy and soya alternatives are offered for every recipe.

Overweight, underweight or just right?

Children and adults who are allergic to wheat, dairy, soya or nuts can still be overweight or underweight, neither of which is healthy for them.

On the one hand, a person who has been losing weight due to vomiting, diarrhoea or feeling too uncomfortable to eat may quickly re-gain a healthy weight once the problem foods are eliminated from their diet, and their symptoms disappear.

21

You should know whether a member of your family is underweight or overweight just by looking at them. A table of weight-to-height or age ratios may appear to give a scientific standard by which to measure your child but, in fact, these can be unhelpful. For example, the baby weight charts given out by many health visitors are based on averages for bottle-fed babies who tend to gain weight more quickly than breast-fed infants. These charts do not allow for racial differences or any other inherited genetic tendencies that your child has towards a particular growth pattern. For this reason we do not include height/weight tables in this book.

Instead, if possible the whole family needs to take a serious and supportive look at each other. If a member looks thin, and you can see their ribs and other bones beneath their skin then they are underweight. They need to increase their calorie intake in a healthy way. However, if a family member has a chubby face and body with rolls of fat round their stomach and easily gets overheated and starts panting after a few minutes running around, then they are overweight. They need to eat more fruit and vegetables, cut their supply of crisps, sweets, biscuits, cakes, fried food, pizzas and take-aways and get into the habit of doing more exercise.

Of course as parents, it can be easier not to look honestly at our child's size because it may reflect on our own body shape. Denying your child is overweight and calling them 'well covered', rather than accepting they are obese and that therefore you are too, may be easier but accepting the reality could help the whole family towards a longer, fitter life. If you are in any doubt as to whether your children or you are a healthy weight consult your doctor.

If your child falls into neither category, just be aware of lifestyle changes that might mean that they are likely to become too fat or too thin and change their diet accordingly. For example, up until now your son has eaten a lot of high energy foods but played a lot of football – now he is getting obsessed with computer games and so exercising less but he still continues eating the same. He is likely to start gaining weight unless you help him change his diet.

Trying to encourage everyone in your family to take regular exercise is an important part of keeping everyone fit and helping them to maintain a healthy body weight. Even 30 minutes exercise every day has benefits. Finding the time can seem difficult but some of these suggestions may help. The important thing is to try to enjoy whatever you choose to do. Making exercise part of your quality family time together helps the parents become good role models for the children, helps you to have fun, and hopefully, will build a bank of happy memories to look back on in later years. You could try:

- walking to school, or even parking further away from the gates and walking the last part of the journey

- parking further away from the shops, cinema or café you are about to visit rather than as close as you can possibly get so that you build in some walking

- going for a walk in the woods, or along the beach (taking a picnic, even in winter, adds to the fun)

- playing football at the local park, or throwing a ball or Frisbee, playing family rounders or cricket

- swimming, riding bikes, scooters or roller-skating

- having a dance mat, Wii or Eye Toy competition on days when you can't get out.

Children's changing nutritional needs

Growing children need to increase their intake of calories, protein, vitamins and minerals such as calcium when they go through growth spurts. However, it is not just as children grow that their nutritional needs change. Children who previously spent much of their time running around need fewer calories when they change interests and spend their free-time standing around chatting or slumped in front of the television, computer or games console.

Your child's mood can affect their appetite. In general, happy children are more likely to eat when they are hungry and to refuse food if they are not. Helping a happy child to eat the right proportions of different foods and ensuring that they are not constantly munching foods that are high in sugars or refined carbohydrates will allow their appetites to dictate a healthy input of food.

In contrast, a child who is often over-tired or feeling miserable may not feel like eating or, alternatively, may comfort eat. After helping such a child to deal with the underlying causes, eating a healthy diet free from allergens to which she is sensitive which contains a higher proportion of foods that have a low GI index should help to lift moods and help to re-balance the appetite.

A 'special diet'

Your heart may be sinking as you think of a family member's life being restricted by the need to follow a 'special diet'. However, the reality is that we all follow special diets to some degree because we limit our food shopping according to what is available, our culture, personal taste, and our budget. The benefit to your family member in following their particular special diet is enormous. Not only does it avoid making them ill, but it may be easier to ensure that they follow a healthy diet since they will be unable to eat the additive-loaded, highly processed foods that scientists believe cause a great deal of ill health. Using the recipes in this book can help you to ensure that the food your family shares is tasty, additive-free and rich in vitamins and minerals.

Health benefits for the other family members

Everyone in the family can enjoy the benefits of a healthy, varied diet while reducing the amount they consume of wheat, dairy, soya and nuts. Non-allergic members of the family who are fed from the recipes in this book while continuing to eat wheat, dairy, soya and nuts at other times are likely to be eating a much wider range of foods than they have before. By eating a more varied diet we give our bodies a better chance of taking in the full range of vitamins and trace minerals.

Since there is a genetic tendency towards wheat and milk intolerance many scientific communities advocate delaying the introduction of highly allergenic foods into the diet of children coming from such a background. Couple this with health concerns about the presence of nuts and soya in so much processed food and, by feeding the rest of your family these recipes, you may be protecting their health.

This is good news for the person preparing meals, as you can save time and effort by passing on the health-giving benefits of 'the restricted diet' and feed the whole family the same delicious meals. Initially your child may whinge a little at the changes in diet, but, happily, we have found that there are three inescapable truths when it comes to feeding growing children:

1) If they are properly hungry, then children learn to eat what is available if it is tasty, even if they moan at first.

2) Given the opportunity to change, children come to prefer eating 'real' tasty food rather than bland 'junk'.

3) Not offering any other choice of food and removing all the banned foods from your cupboards makes winning the battle easier. No one can eat what is not there.

Having experienced the demands of feeding a family where not everyone shares the same restricted diet, we have developed the recipes with this in mind.

In whatever way you choose to cook for your family – one recipe for all or two versions of the same dish – by sharing the meal and treating it as normal fare for everyone, a potential source of conflict is eliminated. It is not a case of comparing 'your special food' and 'my ordinary food' – rather we all eat 'our yummy food' and enjoy mealtimes together without anyone feeling they are less or more favoured.

Summary

- Everyone benefits from eating a healthy diet rather than one loaded with refined, processed foods that are high in fats and calories but low in vitamins and minerals.

- Giving the whole family the same allergen-free food reduces meal-time stress for the cook!

- It is possible to eat a healthy diet while avoiding wheat, dairy, soya and nuts, but non-intolerant family members can continue to enjoy the sufferer's problem foods at other times when the whole family is not eating together.

4: Shopping to avoid Wheat, Dairy, Soya and Nuts

If only avoiding putting any dairy in your trolley was as simple as just not buying any milk, cheese, yoghurt or butter. But ingredients such as wheat, milk, soya, and nuts are the unexpected ingredient in an enormous number of foods. In fact you may find it impossible to buy ready prepared meals if a member of your family needs to eliminate more than one of these key foods. Whatever diet restrictions you have to live with, reading the ingredients listed on the label or packaging of any ready-processed food or ready-prepared meal has to become second nature if you are to avoid certain ingredients.

Since 2004 a European law has stipulated the clear labelling of these 14 ingredients:
milk,
eggs,
peanuts,
nuts from trees (including Brazil nuts, hazelnuts, almonds and walnuts)
fish,
crustaceans (including crab and shrimps)
soya,
wheat,
celery,
mustard,
sesame,
sulphur dioxide,
lupin flour,
molluscs.

In response to this, many manufacturers print brightly coloured Allergy Alert or information boxes on their packaging, stating which of the 14 foods are present. However, recent surveys show that some companies are still not complying with the law, so it is always wise to check the list of ingredients. There are also anomalies. For example, the Food Standards Agency states that soya oil does not have to be labelled individually when used in blended vegetable oil because refined soya oil 'should be safe' for people with soya allergy. Milk and wheat may be used as clarifying agents for wine and then not included as ingredients. (An additional concern is that milk is used in some washing-up liquids and to lubricate machines producing latex but its presence in these products does not have to be stated by manufacturers).

Since ingredients may be included under a variety of names the lists in the table on the next page will help you to decipher the ingredients on most items. Having said that, the list below cannot be exhaustive, so the safest rule is: 'if in doubt, don't buy'. After all, you can always cook something else for dinner and phone the manufacturer on their customer care-line to check the ingredients before your next shopping trip.

If you are already familiar with the way foods are labelled and have scoured your supermarket shelves looking for ready produced foods that the member(s) of the family requiring a restricted diet can eat, you will know how disheartening this can be. Although there is a growing range of wheat-free, dairy-free, soya-free and nut-free items to choose from, it is still difficult to find products that enable you to avoid a combination of ingredients, foods that are not loaded with additives and preservatives, that still taste good and are not frighteningly expensive.

These drawbacks usually ensure that feeding these items to the whole family remains an unrealistic option. For these and other reasons, home-baking soon becomes the best choice. With this in mind we have prepared the following advice on the basic ingredients used in our recipes, all of which you can find in the major supermarkets.

Some alternative ingredient names:

Wheat	Milk	Soya	Nuts
flour, gluten, cereal, binder, binding, cereal filler, cereal protein, cereal starch, edible starch, food starch, modified starch, wholegrain, binder, vegetable protein, thickening or thickener, rusk, fructose derived from wheat.	milk, cheese, cream, sour cream, crème fraiche, buttermilk, smetaa, fromage frais, yoghurt, butter, butterfat, whey, casein, caseinate, hydrolysed casein, albumin, albumen, lactoalbumin, lactic acid, lactose, non fat milk solids, skimmed milk powder, lacto globulin.	soya beans, soya gum, soya flour, lecithin, vegetable gum, hydrolysed vegetable protein, soy protein isolate, protein concentrate, textured vegetable protein TVP, vegetable starch, bean curd, tofu, vegetable oil (simple, fully or partially hydrogen-ated), plant sterols.	*Although there are no common synonyms for other nuts, these names are used for* **peanuts:** Ground-nut, groundnut oil, peanut oil, vegetable oil, arachis oil.

Alternatives to wheat products

In recent years supermarkets have begun to stock a wider variety of non-wheat flours as listed below. The specialised blends are considerably more expensive than their wheat counterparts, but the single-ingredient flours used in many of the recipes in this book are considerably cheaper than those blends. The specialised blends and rice flours have a high glycaemic index (as, of course, does refined white flour) but gram flour, buckwheat flour and cornmeal (polenta) have a lower glycaemic index and are also higher in fibre.

Since it is a real challenge to produce tasty gluten-free food, it helps if you can keep the full range of flours in your kitchen cupboard in order to vary your family's diet.

Flour alternatives

Not all the non-wheat flours are suitable for Coeliacs but many of the ones included below are. It is worth being aware that supermarkets sell many of the single-ingredient flours listed below in more than one place:

1) in the home-baking section

2) in the allergy/special diet section where these flours are usually found in 1kg bags;

3) on the shelf providing cooking ingredients for specific ethnic groups where these flours are sold in larger quantities and at a cheaper price.

Gluten-free bread flours are made from a blend of non-wheat flours such as rice, potato and tapioca with xanthan gum added to compensate for the missing gluten needed in bread-making that ensures that your loaf will still rise. At the moment there are no brown bread flour alternatives readily available in supermarkets. If you follow the recipe on p85 you will be able to bake your own by using buckwheat flour.

Gluten-free plain flour is made from a blend of non-wheat flours such as rice flour, potato flour, tapioca flour, maize flour, sarrasin flour, etc. It is a lot more expensive than the wheat version. Although this blended flour is designed to be used for all general baking purposes, it has different cooking properties to conventional flour: (see p43-44). This needs to be borne in mind when you are cooking or it is easy to produce very unappetising results.

In a similar way to refined white wheat flour, these gluten-free blends have a high GI index, which when combined with sugar in cakes, puddings or biscuits can quickly set off the high/low blood sugar swings. For all these reasons many of the recipes in this book often use the single-ingredient flours listed below.

Rice flour is a gluten-free fine flour made from a mix of white and brown rice. Although ground rice is similar and cheaper to buy, it is much coarser in texture. Unless your blender or food processor can mill it to produce the light flour needed for baking, it is best to stick to the rice flour.

Gram flour (also called besam flour) is a gluten-free flour made from a variety of finely ground chick pea which means that it is relatively high in protein and fibre. **It is important to remember that gram flour is unsuitable for children and adults whose nut allergy means that they also need to avoid legumes.** The flour is pale yellow and has a distinctively nutty flavour. Traditionally it has been used for savoury dishes or nut-enriched sweetmeats in Asian cooking. However, we have discovered that gram flour can also be used to make delicious cake (p222), home-made pasta (p130), ham and sweetcorn fritters (p102) and onion bhajias (p106).

Buckwheat flour (or sarrassin flour) comes from a plant that is a member of the rhubarb family and is a sweet, light brown, gluten-free flour traditionally used for making crepes in France, noodles in northern China, and blinis in Russia. Its colour and taste also make it an excellent basis for recipes such as our basic bread (p86) and toddler birthday chocolate cake (p80). This flour has a higher fibre content than some of the other flours.

Cornmeal (polenta) is pale yellow in colour and made from ground maize (sweet corn). It contains some gluten and is useful for making tortillas, pizza bases, coating for fish or chicken nuggets, cakes and puddings and can also be used as a thickener.

Oat flour is not always available in supermarkets, however, a sufficiently fine flour can be achieved by whizzing rolled porridge oats in a food processor or blender. If you need to buy gluten free foods it is very difficult to buy oats that have not been contaminated with wheat or barley so make sure you really have purchased completely pure oats before grinding them.

If you are not on a wheat-free diet then the supermarket own-brand economy-packaged oats are usually smaller and finer than the top-grade branded alternatives which means that they cook to a softer texture much more quickly.

Oat flour is used in the oat biscuits recipe (p212) and can also be used as a thickener. (Plain oats and oatmeal are also useful ingredients for making porridge, flapjacks and crumble toppings.)

Oats contain are a valuable source of both soluble and insoluble fibre.

Pasta alternatives

Most of the big supermarkets now sell wheat-free pasta shapes made from rice, millet or corn. Some have even begun to produce their own brands but it is important to check the list of ingredients on these as they are usually made from a blend of flours and often include soya flour.

The variety of shapes available may be limited so making your own can give you more variety. If you want flat sheets of pasta to make lasagne, cannelloni or ravioli then try the simple recipe for pasta dough on p130. If you own (or can borrow) a pasta machine, the same dough can be used to make a more interesting variety of pasta shapes.

Couscous alternatives

Among some supermarkets' specialist foods ranges can be found the *Berlize* brand of barley couscous which is a tasty alternative to the wheat version. It cooks the same as the wheat variety and has the same light, fluffy texture. Perhaps more importantly, barley couscous, like wheat couscous, is very quick to cook – you just place the desired quantity in a heat-proof bowl, pour on enough boiling water to cover it and leave for a few minutes until the grain has swelled.

Barley does contain gluten and so it is not suitable for those on a gluten-free diet, for example, Coeliacs.

Alternatives to dairy products

Dairy products are: cow's milk, cream, crème fraiche, smetna, sour cream, fromage frais, butter, butter milk, cheese and yoghurt.

Some children who are intolerant to cow's milk products are better able to tolerate goat, sheep or buffalo milk products but the protein structure of these is still very similar to cow's milk and so for many people complete avoidance of all animal milks is the best solution.

Milk alternatives

There are three main plant-based milk alternatives readily available from supermarkets and can be used for the recipes in this book:

- rice milk fortified with calcium - a blander, thin, white sweet milk.
- oat milk - pale yellow, richer than rice milk and with a distinctive oat flavour.
- soya milk: pale yellow and creamy, it can be purchased unsweetened with a distinctively beany taste or ready sweetened with apple juice.

N.B. An allergy to soya-protein has been found to co-exist with an allergy to the cow's milk protein in a significant number of cases (and in some cases to peanut allergy too). In these cases the use of soya milk as an alternative to cow's milk is not appropriate.

The table on the next page allows you to compare the different nutritional contents of cow's milk and fortified rice, soya and oat milk. Their different cooking qualities are discussed in chapter 5.

Comparison of nutritional content of milk alternatives

Typical values: per 100ml	Cow's milk (full fat)	Soya milk (un-sweet ened)	Rice Milk (fortified)	Oat milk (fortified)
energy	250kj 60kcal	134 kj 32 kcal	209kj 50kcal	180kj 45kcal
protein	3.2g	3.4g	0.1g	1g
carbo-hydrate	5.2g	0.2g	9.6g	6.5g
fat saturated unsaturated	3.25g 1.9g 1.35g	1.8g 0.3g 1.5g	1.2g 0.2g 1.0g	1.5g 0.2g 1.3g
fibre		0.6g	0.0g	0.8g
sodium		trace	0.03g	0.05g
Vitamins % RDA	A 3% B1 3% B2 12% B12 18% D 20%	E 15% B2 15% D 15% B12 50%	A 15% D2 15%	D 10% B2 10% Folic acid 10% B12 20%
Minerals % RDA	Calcium 11% Magne-sium 3% Potassi-um 3%	Calcium 15%	Calcium 15%	Calcium 15%

RDA = UK Recommended Daily Allowance

Butter alternatives

At the time of writing it is hard to find margarine that does not contain any milk products at all and very difficult to find ones that are both non-dairy and non-soya. If you experience difficulties in finding a dairy-free and/or soya-free margarine contact the supermarket's customer care-line to check what is included in the ingredients, especially as manufacturers do not have to declare using soya oil in a blended vegetable oil. Even after you have found a margarine that suits your needs, it is still wise to keep checking the ingredient list as recipes can be changed without notice. A margarine called *Pure* which is dairy-free and based on sunflower oil is available at the larger supermarkets and there are several varieties, including one that is entirely dairy and soya free.
Goat's butter is available in some supermarkets.

Cheese alternatives

Sheep, goat and buffalo cheeses are readily available in supermarkets as an alternative to dairy cheese if your child can tolerate them. There is also a range of soya* cheese and rice milk cheeses available from some larger supermarkets but you still need to check their labels as dairy ingredients are sometimes included. These cheese alternatives can be eaten in salads, sandwiches, etc., as well as being used in the recipes in this book.

(see page 35 for information about situations when soya is not a suitable alternative to cow's milk.)*

Yoghurt and cream alternatives

Sheep and goat yoghurt and goat's cream can be found in large supermarkets. Oat cream is becoming more widely available. Currently there are no rice milk alternatives to yoghurt or cream. Soya* yoghurt is available and there is also a cream alternative (*Soya Dream* is the most frequently available brand). Coconut cream is another cream option but its distinctive flavour may not suit all recipes.

Ice-cream alternatives

Dairy-free sorbets are sometimes available in supermarkets, while oat milk ice-cream is only occasionally available. Soya milk* alternatives to dairy ice-cream are more readily available. The range of flavours is still limited and the list of ingredients and additives included may encourage you to try making your own. A recipe for delicious home-made (and additive free!) ice-cream (with suggestions for numerous flavour variations) can be found on p182.

Chocolate

Buying the best quality, high cocoa content plain chocolate available will usually ensure that the chocolate is dairy-free. However, it may still contain soya lecithin, and the manufacturer may be unwilling to guarantee that the product is entirely nut free if it is produced in the same factory as the company's nut chocolate variety.
Cocoa powder is naturally free from wheat, dairy and soya and nuts.

(*see page 35 for information about when soya is not a suitable alternative to milk.)

Other useful ingredients

To add variety and compensate for the exclusion of wheat, dairy and soya, we have found these store-cupboard staples invaluable:
cornflakes
rice crispies
potato
cornflour
quinoa
barley
rice
vanilla extract
lemon
fresh, dried herbs and spices such as: cinnamon, nutmeg and ginger.

Summary

- Shopping for a member of the family who has food allergies requires careful reading of ingredient lists although the Allergy Alert information box on most packaging is now making this a lot easier.

- Many processed foods and ready-made meals contain hidden wheat, milk or soya. Cooking your own dishes can quickly become the easiest option to avoid including unwanted ingredients in your family's diet.

- Larger supermarkets often stock the alternative flours and milks you will need in unexpected places and at varying prices. Some careful shopping will keep the cost down!

5: Cooking tips

The three sections in this chapter will help you to get the most out of the recipes in this book and help to make sure that you can cook for your family while continuing to manage a busy lifestyle.

Managing your kitchen:

- **Store** all dry ingredients in sealed plastic containers in store cupboards to prevent cross-contaminations of non-allergen foods by allergen-containing food.

- **Weigh** the ingredients carefully even after you have been cooking a recipe for a while. It is especially important to get the dry ingredient-to-liquid ingredient ratios right when you are using gluten-free flours or the end result becomes too dry and crumbly. Spoon measurements are for level spoonfuls.

- **Oven** temperatures in this book are based on fan-assisted ovens which are hotter and faster than traditional ovens. If you have a traditional oven you will need to increase the temperature by 10C to 20C. Always consult your manufacturer's guide for information.

- **Cooking times** may vary as a result of the type of oven used.

- **Cake tin sizes** make a big difference to how long and at what temperature a cake should be cooked. For this reason all the recipes in the book specify a particular size tin.

- **Olive oil** not extra virgin olive oil is used in recipes unless they specifically state otherwise. Check that your oil is not blended with nut oils or sesame oil.

- **Soak** fresh fruit and vegetables in cold water for at least an hour to remove pesticides, moulds, etc., before using them.

- **Fry** allergen-free foods in fresh cooking oil, and fry before food containing the allergens you are avoiding.
- **Clean** your equipment, utensils, work surfaces and oven carefully before cooking allergen-free food.
- **Prepare** and cook the allergen-free food first to avoid cross-contamination as even a trace of dairy, gluten, nuts or soya can make some people very ill.
- **Check** you have all the ingredients before you start cooking since it is not easy to make last-minute substitutions when you have to use wheat-free, dairy-free or soya-free ingredients.
- **Label** allergen-free food carefully before storing it.
- **Be aware** of how much time you have to cook before you start – some recipes have more stages than others. (Hungry children needing dinner will give you much less hassle if you choose a quick and easy recipe!)
- **Learning to cook** is a vital skill for children who will continue having to live with a restricted diet for many years.
- **Young children** love helping with meal preparation so try to make cooking time an enjoyable family occasion. At first, children will need a lot of supervision but even the youngest can put vegetable peelings in the recycling bin, collect ingredients from the cupboard, peel off the outer skin of an onion or pull off leaves from cabbages and lettuces.
- **Older children** enjoy helping to operate the food mixer and can even learn some basic maths while they help with measuring, weighing and timing.
- **Young chefs** may want to graduate to attempting whole recipes. With this in mind we have included a section of easy recipes for older children to cook (p224-241).

Advice on using alternative ingredients

Dairy alternatives:

Oat milk

This is a good alternative to cow's milk or soya. The carton needs shaking well before use each time to make sure the milk is a good consistency because it can separate. When the carton is 'empty' try swilling it out with 100ml of cold water and you'll have another 100mls of oat milk to use. Oat milk is really creamy tasting (it makes delicious porridge) and is an enjoyable cold drink.

Oat cream

This is a rich cream that tastes delicious – it is nice just poured over fresh fruit and it works well in both savoury and sweet recipes. Although it does not whip, it enriches desserts, custards and sauces and can be set with gelatine.

Rice milk

This is the most non-allergenic milk. It has a watery, thin consistency and tends to deliver less creamy results in recipes (which is one reason why it is more easily digested). It works well in both sweet and savoury dishes. Unflavoured rice milk is used in all the recipes but the flavoured variety is a refreshing drink.

Soya milk*

Soya milk is similar to cow's milk in consistency, has a distinctive (but not unpleasant) flavour and cooks well in sweet and savoury dishes. It can curdle when added to acidic or hot ingredients, e.g., for example when added to hot coffee.

(* see page 35 for information about when soya is not a suitable alternative to cow's milk.)

Soya cream*

This is a good alternative to pouring cream and although it does not whip it enriches desserts, custards and sauces. Soya cream can be thickened with gelatine to become mousse-like.

Soya cheese*

This melts well in sauces and melts and becomes crisp when used as a topping. It can also be eaten plain with crackers or in sandwiches.
(see page 35 for information about when soya is not a suitable alternative to cow's milk.)*

Wheat and/or gluten-free alternatives

Gluten-free plain flour (Usually made from a blend of rice, potato, tapioca, maize and sarrasin flour.)

This is a good substitute for plain flour and works well in sauces and batters. You will need to use more liquid and baking powder in recipes to get similar results to wheat flour. Used on its own, biscuits and cakes made with gluten-free flour have a drier, crumbly and denser texture, and leave a dry 'clartie' taste in your mouth afterwards. They are lighter in colour than those made with wheat flour. The recipes in this book have been developed to overcome these problems.

Gluten-free bread flour (Usually made from a blend of rice, potato and tapioca flours mixed with xanthan gum)

This blend of flour makes a dense, heavy loaf. The texture and taste improves if you use half gluten-free bread flour and half buckwheat flour. Adding extra xanthan gum and a beaten egg also helps to improve the texture of the bread. (For more information on bread-making, see p85)

Buckwheat or sarrasin flour.

This cooks well on its own or blended with other flours. It has a distinctive nutty flavour and is popular in European cooking for making pancakes (galettes and blinis). It adds a brown 'wholemeal' type colour to recipes, and like other gluten-free flour recipes absorbs more liquid and needs more raising agent than wheat.

Rice flour

Used alone this adds a grainy texture to cakes and biscuits but this is not noticeable when it is used in chocolate brownies. It works well combined with gluten-free flour to make shortbread biscuits or cakes and with maize flour to make cakes. Like other gluten-free flours, rice flour needs more liquid and baking agents to get results similar to those with wheat flour.

Cornmeal flour or polenta

This coarse, yellow flour adds a lovely sunshine yellow hue to dishes. It has a grainy texture and a faint, distinctive flavour which is pleasant in savoury dishes but easily masked in cakes and biscuits. It works well coating chicken or fish for 'nuggets', in pizza bases and in cakes. Polenta (baked or fried) can be served with casseroles as an alternative to mashed potatoes or pasta.

Gram flour *(not suitable for people with allergy to legumes)*

This yellow flour has a strong 'nutty' distinctive flavour which works best with spices in cakes or savoury dishes such as fritters and onion bhajias. Its high-fibre content can help to lower the glycaemic index of dishes. Gram flour requires more liquid and raising agents than wheat flour. It is not suited to bread or cooking with yeast.

Quinoa (pronounced 'keenwha')

This is a coarse grain that is a delicious alternative to bulgar wheat or couscous. It can be added to soups, eaten cold as part of a salad or served hot with a casserole.

Oats

Oats contain a similar protein to gluten and some Coeliacs are unable to eat them. Rolled oats are useful for coating meat or fish, thickening sauces, adding to biscuits or crumble mixtures. Their presence can lower the glycaemic index of a dish. **If you need to eat a wheat-free diet make sure that the oats you buy are not contaminated with wheat.**

Gluten-free baking powder

This works in the same way and in the same quantities as traditional baking powder.

Gluten-free stock cubes

These are widely available and you may prefer to use them in all your cooking as their ingredients seem to be more natural than the stock cubes containing wheat. However, they do tend to have a saltier taste. Making your own stock is relatively easy but can be time-consuming. If you do make your own stock, it is worth producing large batches, then freezing in small freezer bags.

Soy sauce*

Gluten-free soy sauce can be used in the same way as the version containing wheat.

(* see page 35 for information about when soya is not a suitable alternative to cow's milk.)

Chocolate

For a wheat-free or gluten-free diet white, milk or plain chocolate can be used in recipes. For dairy-free recipes only 70% plain chocolate (or darker) can be used. (Not all plain chocolate is dairy-free). Soya lecithin is the emulsifier in some chocolate but plain chocolate that does not include it can be found in most supermarkets.

Vanilla

Always use a good quality real vanilla extract such as *Bourbon Madagascar* because the vanilla flavour is much more intense. Vanilla is especially useful when you need to mask the intensity of soya's taste, if that is your choice of milk, and is invaluable in helping you to achieve the best results if you cook gluten-free.

Labour and time-saving equipment

Even though every task in the kitchen can be done using simple equipment, electrical devices can save lots of time and do, often, produce better results. However, since it is possible to buy a gadget for almost every job it is important to know how to choose the ones that really will make cooking dishes for a restricted diet better, faster and more enjoyable.

Food mixer

Mixers are best for stirring, beating and whisking ingredients. They cope well with family-sized quantities, especially cake mixtures, and can be operated slowly so ingredients are carefully incorporated and not over-processed. There are two types: free-standing and hand-held.

Hand-held mixers are very compact, cheap to buy, easy to store, can be used with any bowl or jug and only the beaters need cleaning at the end of cooking.

A table-top mixer takes up space in the kitchen but is a worthwhile investment especially if you can have it out ready-to use and are committed to cooking regularly.

Food processor

A multi-purpose machine that is ideal for chopping, grinding, grating, slicing, shredding, mixing and puréeing. If you have more than one vegetable to chop, grate or purée it is worth using the food processor as, in a matter of seconds, even large quantities of vegetables can be rapidly prepared. Whole blocks of cheese can be grated quickly using a food processor and then stored in a resealable plastic food bag in the fridge ready for use.

Food processors can be used to blend soups, make purées and prepare larger quantities of baby foods but generally the results are not as smooth as those achieved with a blender or hand-held blender.

When making a cake in a food processor it is a good idea to leave the filler chute open so that as much air as possible is incorporated into the mixture.

Food blender

Blenders are great for making smoothies, purées, soups and baby foods. Some models can cope with dry ingredients so that you can make bread or biscuit crumbs, or chop fresh herbs in them. If you are choosing a table-top model, make sure the controls are simple, and the jug holds more than a litre in capacity, has a handle, is robust and preferably dishwasher proof.

Hand blenders are particularly useful for puréeing or making soups because they can be placed into any bowl, jug or saucepan. They are easy to clean and are readily stored in a drawer or cupboard.

If you are going to be preparing baby or toddler food regularly, then a blender is essential.

Bread-maker

Using a machine to mix and knead dough makes the process a lot easier, and saves time. If you are going to have to make bread regularly for family members on a restricted diet then a bread-maker is indispensable and the rest of the family can enjoy delicious home-made wheat bread while you enjoy knowing exactly what ingredients it contains.

Although a food mixer with a dough hook can mix bread dough efficiently, the whole process is still very labour-intensive. With a bread-maker all you have to do is place the paddle in the tin, place the ingredients in it, choose the right menu and start the machine. Most models will even allow you to set a timer so that you can wake up to the smell of a freshly baked loaf!

Microwave oven

Some people use their microwave oven to cook everything; for others it is a supplement. However, it certainly helps families with restricted diets as batches of food can be frozen and then de-frosted and heated quickly on days when you are too busy to cook a meal for them or everyone else is having a take-away.

Ice-cream maker

This machine is only worth buying if the family member on a dairy-free diet eats a lot of ice-cream. Non dairy ice-cream is not always readily available and can be expensive so an ice-cream maker can make life more enjoyable and recoup its cost over time.

Slow cooker

Slow cookers are a great way for busy people to prepare family meals in advance during the winter months. You can prepare the food in the morning or, if you prefer, get everything ready the night before and refrigerate it overnight. Before you leave the house, place the ingredients in the slow cooker and switch it on.

Then, whether people want to eat at 5, 6, or 8 o' clock their dinner is ready and it won't have dried out or burnt. Bolognese, curry, casseroles and milk puddings are all delicious cooked in this way and any portions that are left over can be cooled and frozen as a healthy ready-meal.

If you are buying a slow cooker, choose one that is a large family-size and has a removable bowl for easy washing up. Make sure that the cooker has a setting that brings the food to the boil before it turns down to simmer.

Beginning to use new ingredients, recipes and pieces of equipment may seem a little daunting at first but in a surprisingly short time you will become familiar with them. Seeing the improvement in quality of your family's life will make all your efforts feel worthwhile.

Summary

- Alternative ingredients can behave very differently to their counterparts so follow the recipes exactly!

- Busy cooks can save a lot of time and effort by investing in some key pieces of equipment.

6: Smooth spoonfuls

Currently the World Health Organisation recommends that **weaning** should not begin until an infant is six months old. By this time you may have already tried formula and discovered that your child is allergic to cow's milk and been prescribed one of the **hydrolysed cow's milk** alternatives. These can be used in cooking in the same way that breast milk or formula milk is used: to mix with baby rice or to thin down purées.

Occasionally babies who are allergic to cow's milk cannot tolerate hydrolysed cow's milk either. The flavour of hydrolysed cow's milk is strong and savoury (very different from regular formula and the sweet taste of breast milk). As a result you may find that even after you have persevered your baby refuses to take it or to eat foods that contain it. Whatever your situation, the dietician will help you to ensure that your baby is getting all the vitamins and minerals required by analysing your baby's diet and requesting that your doctor prescribe supplements.

Rice milk can be used to blend baby rice, rice porridge and to thin down vegetable purées, and is generally well tolerated by infants who are allergic to cow's milk or soya. Providing your child is not a coeliac, then **oat milk** is another alternative milk that is very useful in cooking. When using either of these milks you need to bear in mind that:
- rice and oat milks contain little protein
- it is important to choose a brand of oat or rice milk that has been fortified with calcium and vitamins.

Your dietician will advise you as to which milk to use for your baby's earliest solid foods and suggest when you can try introducing soya milk, although the Food Standards

Agency does not recommend that infants are fed soya milk. Like many parents, you may also have concerns about the wisdom of including soya in your child's diet. Eventually rice or oat milk may become your child's staple milk, but this is not recommended before the child is 2 years of age. If so, you will have to ensure that your child consumes adequate amounts of protein, calcium, etc., in other ways.

If you discover that your child is allergic to, or intolerant of, wheat, then your dietician will recommend avoiding wheat and all wheat products. The dietician will suggest alternative cereals that you can use depending on whether your child is a Coeliac or just has an allergy or intolerance. (See Chapter 4 for more information.)

If your baby is unable to tolerate dairy, wheat and/or soya, then initially the dietician is likely to recommend that you avoid giving your infant **egg, fish and nuts** as well. It is also quite common for children with these allergies to be more sensitive to other foods as well and they may not tolerate acidic fruits such as citrus fruits well either. With this in mind the recipes in this section avoid any of these common allergens.

Although trying to work out what your child can have may seem like a culinary nightmare, the good news is that children with allergies usually end up eating a more nutritionally complete diet than their peers. Another positive fact to bear in mind is that the majority of children's problems disappear before they reach five years old. It is rare for a child to start school still needing to follow a very restricted diet although a minority of children do remain allergic to one or more foods.

The following pages offer some simple recipes to help you to get your infant started on the road to healthy and happy eating despite any allergies.

Preparing purées

When you start feeding your baby solids, make sure you try only one food at a time so that if she has a reaction you will know what caused it. Once you are confident that she is able to tolerate a range of fruit and vegetables, you can make her diet more interesting by combining them.

Raw fruit purée

Try ripe:
banana
mango
melon
peaches
pears

These fruits are useful, take-anywhere, instant meals for your baby.

Method

1) Wash the fruit thoroughly, then peel and remove the stone or seeds

2) Mash the fruit with a fork

3) If necessary, use an electric blender, hand-held blender or food processor to blend to the desired consistency with a little of your chosen milk, before serving.

Cooked vegetable and fruit purées

Most babies prefer blander, sweeter tastes initially, so
fruit and root vegetable purées are a good first choice.
apple
asparagus
butternut squash
green beans
broccoli
carrots
cauliflower
courgette
parsnips
potato
swede
sweet potatoes
turnip

Method

1) Wash all fruits or vegetables thoroughly. Then
   carefully peel and remove any seeds or stones.

2) Chop into small pieces, place in a small saucepan and
   cover with water. Bring to the boil and simmer until
   tender for about 10 minutes. *(Alternatively you can cook
   the vegetables in the microwave or steam them.)*

3) Test that the vegetables or fruit are soft, then drain,
   while retaining the cooking water.

4) Mash or blend the cooked fruit or vegetables using an
   electric blender, hand-held blender or food processor
   and adding a little of the cooking water or a suitable
   milk until the purée is the desired consistency. (When
   your child is able to enjoy a thicker texture either
   reduce the amount of cooking water or milk you add,
   or mix in a little baby rice.)

53

5) Check the purée is not too hot before serving. (Test its temperature by dropping a little on your inner wrist – it should feel comfortable.)

6) Any remaining purée you have not served your child can be placed in a clean, covered basin in the fridge or frozen (see below). Throw away any food that remains in the bowl you have been feeding your child from as the saliva that has touched the spoon dipping into it contains many germs.

Freezing purées

Cook and purée the food as described, then cover and leave to cool as quickly as possible. Pour into ice-cube trays and freeze. You can either leave the food in the trays ready to pop out and defrost or, once frozen, tip the cubes into a freezer bag which you have clearly labelled with the name of the food and the date on which you prepared it.

Thawing in the fridge can takes 12-16 hours or it can be done at room temperature over several hours before the food is heated up. Alternatively, you can take the cubes straight out of the freezer and pop in a bowl to cook in the microwave.

After heating the food, stir it carefully and always test its temperature before feeding it to your baby.

Favourite fruit and vegetable combinations

apple and banana
apple and parsnip
apple and pear (and/or peach)
apple and carrot
apricot and pear
apricot and peach
banana and courgette
butternut squash and pear
broccoli and cauliflower
carrot and cauliflower
leek and potato
carrot and swede
carrot and parsnip
potato and parsnip
pea and courgette
sweet potato and apple

Adding more carbohydrate

- Baby rice can be added to a cooked purée (and has the added benefit of being fortified with vitamins and minerals).
- Porridge oats can be added to the pan while the fruit or vegetables are being cooked (provided your child has not been diagnosed as a Coeliac).

Once baby is able to chew try adding these:
- very small pieces of well-cooked rice noodles or wheat-free and/or soya-free pasta.
- cooked rice (glutinous varieties such as Thai or Japanese work best, but any rice will do).

Introducing protein

Once your infant is happily eating vegetables and fruit, you can introduce meat. Since chicken is quite bland this is an easy one to start with, but red meats such as beef or lamb are good as they contain more iron.

Remember:
- all meat needs to be thoroughly cooked.
- introduce one meat for several days so if your child has a reaction you know what caused it.
- meat has a much tougher texture than fruit or vegetables so make it easy to chew by long slow cooking and cutting into tiny chunks or blending.
- Some children with cow's milk allergy may also be allergic to beef.

Although there are some special recipes in this section for babies bear in mind that if a recipe that you prepare for older members of the family does not contain ingredients to which your baby is allergic you may be able to prepare a version for them as follows.

- **Do not add any salt** to the recipes - babies cannot tolerate it.
- put portions of the meat and vegetable parts of your meal into a suitable container.
- add some liquid (water, vegetable cooking water or their milk).
- blend it to a suitable thickness using a blender, hand-held blender or food processor.

7: Toddler tastes

As your child becomes more confident about chewing you can introduce a more varied diet. The following recipes are still free from wheat, dairy, soya, fish and nuts but the last two cake recipes include eggs as your dietician is likely to suggest introducing cooked egg in small proportions. Not only are these cakes popular with small children but the rest of the family will enjoy them too – especially the birthday cake recipe on p80.

Many of the recipes in this section freeze and thaw well so the quantities given are toddler-sized 'one for today and several portions to freeze' to make life easier.

Pre-school is the best time to establish a good pattern of daily eating. A typical day should include three meals and two snacks and might look like this:

Breakfast: Juicy oats(see p60)
Hot chocolate made with soya/rice/oat milk

Snack: Fruity bar (see p76) + water or fruit juice

Lunch: Lamb and sweet potato soup with pasta (see p62)
Piece of carrot cake (see p78) + water or fruit juice

Snack: biscuit (see p196) + soya/rice/oat milk to drink

Dinner: Chicken and thyme rice (see p64) with broccoli, pear and raspberry crumble (see p164)

There is no hard and fast rule about when your child is ready to try the other recipes in this book (puréed to the right consistency). It really is up to you and whether the child can tolerate the other ingredients.

Porridge

A warming breakfast for cold wintry days that is quick enough to make in the microwave so your toddler can enjoy it on weekdays and not just weekends.

Try serving with any of these: a sprinkle of soft brown sugar, honey, golden syrup, jam, fruit purée, sultanas or ½ teaspoon sugar + ½ teaspoon cinnamon.

Serves 1-2

Ingredients

25g porridge oats*
200ml oat, rice or soya milk + extra if needed

Method 1

Place the ingredients in a microwave-proof bowl, stir and then heat on full power for 1 minute, stir again. Then cook for an additional 30 seconds. Add more milk if the porridge is too thick to achieve the desired consistency.

Method 2

Place the ingredients in a small saucepan and place over a medium heat and bring to the boil. Reduce the heat and simmer for 4-5 minutes stirring continually until the oats have softened and the porridge thickened to the desired consistency. Add more milk if the porridge becomes too thick.

* (If your child has to avoid wheat or barley etc. then make sure the oats you buy are completely pure and not contaminated with other cereals.)

Granola

Sweet, crunchy and very more-ish, we find it hard to stop nibbling this cereal – which is why it appears only for special breakfasts and not every day. If you have more self-control then make it regularly, store in an airtight tin and watch your mother-in-law smile when one of your child's first words is a mumbled 'granola'.

Apart from serving it with milk or fruit juice for breakfast, granola can be used as a topping for stewed fruit, sprinkled on ice-cream (see p38), and munched as a snack.

Serves 8-10

Ingredients

250g porridge oats*
50g honey, clear
50g olive oil
100g puréed apple
1 teaspoon cinnamon
150g dried fruit (choose one or a mixture of: sultanas, raisins, blueberries, cherries, chopped apricots, etc.)

Method

1) Pre-heat the oven to 170C/350F/Gas Mark 4.

2) Mix everything except the dried fruit in a large bowl. Then spread the mixture over the base of a roasting tin and place in the oven. Cook for 10 minutes, then stir again. Cook and stir for further 5 minute intervals until the oat mixture is a gentle golden brown – this should take about 25 minutes altogether.

3) Allow to cool. Then stir in the dried fruit. Serve cold.

Juicy Oats

My toddler's favourite breakfast — it still tastes great even if you can only leave it to soak while you are making your child a mug of hot chocolate to enjoy with it to boost their calcium intake. The quantities below make one average toddler-sized portion and can be doubled (or tripled!) to suit your needs.

Serves 1

Ingredients

25g porridge oats*
50ml apple juice, cold
1 tablespoon sultanas,
a few fresh raspberries, strawberries (halved) (optional)

Method

Place the oats, apple juice and sultanas in a bowl. Leave to soak for at least 10 minutes. Stir in the fresh fruit just before serving. Serve cold.

(This can be made the night before and stored in the fridge which makes it refreshingly cool on hot summer mornings.)

(If your child has to avoid wheat or barley etc. then make sure the oats you buy are completely pure and not contaminated with other cereals.)

Chicken and Courgette Soup

An easy soup recipe that can be made from the leftovers from a roast chicken. Serve with bread or turn it into a complete meal by pouring over freshly cooked pasta.

Serves: 8-10 portions

Ingredients

1 onion, peeled and chopped
200g chicken, cooked and diced
2 courgettes, washed and diced
1 large potato, peeled and diced
1-2 tablespoons lemon juice
500ml gluten-free vegetable or chicken stock, hot
2 tablespoons olive oil

Method

1) Fry the onion in the olive oil for 2-3 minutes till softened. Then add the chicken, courgettes, potato, lemon juice and stock.

2) Bring to the boil, then reduce the heat to a simmer for 20 minutes until the vegetables are very soft.

3) Purée the mixture in a blender, food processor or a hand-held blender until smooth. Pour into a clean saucepan and reheat stirring all the time. Check the consistency adding a little more water if it is too thick.

4) Serve hot. Freeze left-overs for another day.

Lamb and Sweet Potato Soup

This protein-rich soup is really useful for lunchtimes and lighter meals. To make it more substantial, serve it with bread (see p86), gnocchi (see p128) or stir in cooked pasta or rice.

Serves 8-10

Ingredients

1 onion, peeled and diced
1 teaspoon dried rosemary
1 tablespoon lemon juice
1 clove garlic, finely chopped
200g lamb, already cooked, diced (e.g. cut from a roast)
400g sweet potato, peeled and diced
500ml gluten-free vegetable stock, hot
2 tablespoons olive oil

Method

1) Place the onion, olive oil, rosemary and garlic in a large saucepan and fry for 2-3 minutes until the onion is softened but not browned. Add the lemon juice and lamb and fry for a further 2-3 minutes.

2) Add the sweet potato and pour in the stock. Bring to the boil and simmer for 20-30 minutes until the sweet potato is soft when pierced with a knife.

3) Purée till it becomes a smooth soup using a blender, food processor or hand-held blender.

4) Serve hot with fresh bread. Freeze leftovers.

Chicken in White Sauce

Chicken in a plain white sauce can form the basis of many simple meals. It is delicious served with rice or pasta but can also be placed in a small dish under any of the toppings described on p69. Try adding ½ teaspoon of dried tarragon or sage to the stock to vary the flavour.

Serves 2-3

Ingredients

1 chicken fillet, washed, diced
15g gluten-free flour
2 tablespoons olive oil
¼ onion peeled, sliced (optional)
75ml gluten-free chicken stock, hot
40ml oat cream or soya cream

Method

1) Place the olive oil in a large frying pan or wok and fry the onion for 2-3 minutes until soft. Add the chicken and fry for 2-3 minutes.

2) Sprinkle the flour over the chicken and onions and stir well. Add the stock and keep stirring to keep the sauce free from lumps. Simmer for 20 minutes until the chicken is cooked through and the sauce has thickened.

3) Reduce the heat and stir in the cream. .

4) Serve hot or cool quickly and refrigerate for the next day.

Chicken and Thyme Rice

A quick and tasty tea-time meal for the whole family. Leftovers can be frozen in ramekin dishes ready for toddler lunches. (Just make sure that there is a good portion of meat in each pot.) If your child dislikes onions then leave them out – it's so much less stressful than watching your child pick out every tiny piece of onion while forgetting to actually eat their meal.

Serves 4-6

Ingredients

200g chicken breast, skinned, diced
200g basmati rice
50g finely chopped broccoli or cauliflower
500ml gluten-free chicken stock, hot
1 teaspoon dried thyme
2 tablespoons lemon juice
2 tablespoons olive oil

Method

1) Heat up the olive oil in a large frying pan and add the chopped onion. Fry over a medium heat for 2-3 minutes until the onion is softened. Then add the diced chicken breast and fry for a further 4-5 minutes. Keep turning the meat over so that every surface is sealed and browned.

2) Reduce the heat, then add the rice, lemon juice and thyme and fry for a further minute stirring continually so that the rice does not stick. Make up the stock with boiling water, and pour over the rice.

3) Add the vegetables and stir well. Continue to cook for a further 5-10 minutes until the rice is cooked. (If all the stock is absorbed before the rice is finished add a little more water.)

4) Serve hot.

Chicken Barley Couscous

Lightly spiced, this dish makes a welcome change from rice and pasta. Barley couscous can be found in the specialist foods section in many supermarkets. (Of course if your toddler can eat wheat, then you can use wheat couscous in this recipe instead.) Barley contains gluten and so cannot be eaten if your child needs to avoid this ingredient (e.g. if they are a Coeliac.)

Serves 4-6

Ingredients

½ onion, peeled, finely chopped
½ teaspoon cumin
½ teaspoon ground coriander
¼ teaspoon ground cinnamon
100g chicken breast, cooked, chopped (or use leftovers from a roast chicken)
200g barley couscous
250ml gluten-free chicken stock, hot
1-2 tablespoons olive oil
25g sultanas

Method

1) In a frying pan, gently fry the onion in the olive oil for 2-3 minutes till softened. Then add the spices and fry for another minute stirring all the time. Add the chicken breast and cook for about five minutes until the chicken is heated through and lightly browned.

2) Make up the stock with boiling water and pour it into the frying pan. Add the sultanas and bring the stock to the boil.

3) Add the couscous and stir gently so that all the ingredients are evenly distributed. Remove the frying pan from the heat and leave it to stand for 5 minutes until the couscous has softened and all the stock has been absorbed.

4) Fluff up with a fork and serve hot with vegetables or cold with salad.

Every-day Mince

Keeping a supply of small dishes two thirds filled with this basic mince mixture in the freezer will mean that you are never short of a ready meal. This mince can be served in a jacket potato or with pasta as a Bolognese sauce or with one of the toppings opposites so your child need never get bored.

Serves 6-8

Ingredients

3 tablespoons olive oil
1 small onion, peeled, finely chopped
1 large carrot, peeled, finely chopped
100g courgettes, washed, finely chopped
250g lean minced beef
2 tablespoon red wine vinegar
300ml gluten-free beef stock, hot
2 teaspoons dried mixed herbs
1x400g tinned chopped tomatoes
1 tube of tomato purée
salt and freshly ground pepper

Method

1) Place the olive oil in a large frying pan or wok. Heat the pan and then add the onion, courgette and carrot. Fry the vegetables to soften them on a high heat for approx. 5 minutes. Stir in the minced beef and red wine vinegar and cook until the beef is lightly browned.

2) Add the stock to the minced beef. Stir well, then add the herbs, tinned tomatoes, tomato purée and seasoning. Stir, cover and simmer for 30 minutes. Purée to desired consistency.

Toppings for every-day mince

Mashed potato

Make a mini shepherd's pie by microwaving a medium-to-large jacket potato. Then scoop out the potato and mashing with a knob of dairy-free &/or soya-free margarine and a tablespoon of your child's usual milk. Top the defrosted mince mixture with the mashed potato. Then either heat through in the oven (180C/375F/Gas Mark 5 for 10 minutes) or microwave for 1 minute until the mince is heated through.

Mashed parsnip and carrot

Peel and dice 1 carrot and 1 parsnip. Cook in boiling water for 15-20 minutes until the vegetables are soft. Drain them then mash together with a knob of dairy-free &/or soya-free margarine. Top the defrosted mince mixture with the mash. Then either heat through in the oven (180C/375F/Gas Mark 5 for 10 minutes) or microwave for 1 minute until the mince is heated through.

Savoury crumble

50g gluten-free flour
Either 25g dairy-free **&/or** soya-free margarine
pinch of mustard powder

Stir the mustard powder and flour together. Then rub in the margarine until the mixture resembles fine bread crumbs. Spoon the crumble mixture over the defrosted mince. Either bake in the oven (180C/375F/Gas Mark 5 for 10 minutes) or microwave for 1-2 minutes until the mince is heated through.

Meatloaf

Slices of meatloaf travel well to parties, other people's homes for lunch and are brilliant pulled out of the freezer and defrosted on busy days. Meatloaf is delicious served with a tomato sauce and mashed potato and broccoli.

Serves 8-10

Ingredients

500g beef mince,
1 onion, peeled, grated
1 apple, peeled, cored, grated
50g porridge oats*
1 tablespoon red wine vinegar
100ml gluten-free beef stock, hot

Method

1) Pre-heat oven to 180C/375F/Gas Mark 5.

2) Place the mince, onion, apple and oats in a mixing bowl and stir well. Pour in the vinegar and stock and mix well.

3) Pour the mixture into the loaf tin, smooth the top. Bake in the oven for 40 minutes then check that the meatloaf is cooked through by piercing with a knife any juices that run out should be clear and the meat should be lightly browned all the way through.

4) Serve hot or cold. (The meatloaf is easier to slice when it is cold.)

(If your child has to avoid wheat or barley etc. then make sure the oats you buy are completely pure and not contaminated with other cerals.)

Mini burgers

Your toddler doesn't have to miss out at barbecues, or when the rest of the family are having a chip and baked beans treat. In fact, you can use the same recipe to make burgers for the whole family rather than using ones bought at the shop, and you have the satisfaction of knowing exactly how they have been made.

Serves 10+

Ingredients

500g minced beef, organic, low fat
½ teaspoon nutmeg
salt and freshly ground pepper

Method

1) Combine all the ingredients together in a mixing bowl.

2) Take large spoonfuls of the mixture and form into round burger shapes using your hands or a burger maker.

3) Pre-heat the grill. Place the burgers on the grill pan rack and cook on a medium setting for approximately 5 minutes before turning over and cooking the other side for a further 5 minutes. Make sure the meat is thoroughly cooked.

4) Serve hot or cold.

Roast Dinner Pots

At first glance this may not seem like much of a recipe but, if your toddler is unable to eat wheat, dairy, soya, nuts, etc. then you are unlikely to be able to feed them any of those standby jars of ready-prepared meals. Keeping a supply of roast dinner pots when your toddler is aged between one and two can be a life saver.

If you need to start cooking this from scratch then place a joint of meat in a roasting tin, surround it with the peeled potatoes and sweet potatoes and roast in the oven for the recommended time at 180C/375F/Gas Mark 5 (see main courses recipes). Cook the broccoli so that it is ready at the same time the roast finishes cooking.

Serves 10+

Ingredients

500g chicken, lamb, beef, roasted and finely chopped
400g potato, cooked
400g sweet potato, cooked
200g broccoli, boiled till soft enough for your child (reserve the cooking water)

Method

1) Place the meat and vegetables in a food processor or blender and blend until the ingredients are fully combined and chopped fine enough to suit your child's chewing power. If necessary add enough of the broccoli cooking water to ensure that the mix is moist enough to suit your child's taste.

2) Serve hot or place in individual small dishes and cool quickly for the next day's meal or freeze.

Pork and Coriander Meatballs

A yummy finger food, these are popular when served with rice and vegetables or mashed potato and baked beans. The quantities below make 20 meatballs and they freeze well once cooked.

Serves 6-8

Ingredients

500g pork mince
1 teaspoon ground coriander
1 clove garlic, crushed
pinch sugar
4 tablespoons olive oil for frying
2 tablespoons polenta

Method

1) Place the pork mince, coriander, garlic and pinch of sugar together in a mixing bowl and stir thoroughly. Take out one tablespoon of the mixture at a time and shape it into small balls using your hands.

2) Sprinkle the polenta onto a piece of kitchen paper on a plate. Roll the meatballs in the polenta to coat them.

3) Pour the olive oil into a large frying pan and heat for 1-2 minutes so that the pan is hot. Gently fry the meatballs in batches for 3-4 minutes until the meat is thoroughly cooked through.

4) When cooked place on a piece of kitchen paper on a plate to allow excess fat to drain off. Serve hot or cold.

Chocolate Pudding

Using the gluten-free flour creates the lightest, most deliciously chocolaty pudding imaginable. Portions wrapped in foil freeze beautifully and travel well. The sight of my toddler's pudding bowl filled with slightly warmed chocolate pudding and icy raspberry sorbet drives me to hover by her high chair, willing her to do the impossible – leave some for me!

Serves 16-20

Ingredients

Either 225g soft butter
          or dairy-free **&/or** soya-free margarine
375 g light muscovado sugar
2 large eggs, beaten
1 teaspoon vanilla extract
100g 70% plain dairy-free and soya-free chocolate, melted
200g gluten-free flour
2 teaspoon bicarbonate of soda
Either 300ml boiling water **or** 300ml boiling oat milk or rice milk

Method

1) Pre-heat the oven to 180C/375F/Gas Mark 5. Grease a 25cm square cake tin.

2) Cream the margarine and sugar, then add the beaten eggs and vanilla and mix well. Stir in the melted chocolate.

3) Add the flour and bicarbonate of soda spoonful by spoonful, alternating with the boiling water or oat or rice milk and keep mixing until you have a very liquid, but smooth batter.

4) Pour into the prepared cake tin. *Half fill a roasting tin with boiling water and place the cake tin into the middle of this. Then bake for 25 minutes until the cake is cooked and a cake skewer comes out clean.

5) Serve warm.

* N.B. Make sure any small children are out of the kitchen when this cake is being placed in the oven.

Fruity Bars

These soft, easy-to-chew fruit and oat bars are ideal for babies and toddlers (and older children will enjoy them as a healthy mid-morning school snack). You can buy similar in the supermarket but these are much more economical. For variety, replace the dried dates with an equal quantity of dried apricots or dates and sultanas.

Makes 12 pieces

Ingredients

200g dried dates, stoned, chopped
200ml cold water or oat milk or rice milk
Either 25g dairy-free **&/or** soya-free margarine
200g porridge oats*
100ml apple juice

(If your child has to avoid wheat or barley etc. then make sure the oats you buy are completely pure and not contaminated with other cerals.)

Method

1) 1 Pre-heat the oven to 150C/325F/Gas Mark 5.

2) Grease an 18 x 23cm rectangular baking dish.

3) Place the dates and water or oat or rice milk in a small pan and bring to the boil. Then simmer for 10 minutes until the dates are soft. (Alternatively place the dates and water in a microwave proof bowl and cook for 5 minutes. Stir, then cook for 2 minutes. Stir again.)

4) Blend the dates and cooking water to a smooth purée. While still hot, stir in the margarine mixing until it is fully blended.

5) Add the oats stirring thoroughly. Pour in the apple juice mix well and leave for a few minutes while the oats soften.

6) Place the mixture in the baking dish and cook for 10 minutes in the pre-heated oven, until firm and slightly golden (or cook on full power for 4 minutes in the microwave until firm and golden). Cool in the tin and cut into squares.

7) Once cooled, these bars can be wrapped in foil and stored in an air tight tin or frozen.

Carrot Cake

Even members of the family who dislike carrots really love this cake – so not only is it moist and delicious but it's a useful way of getting another portion of vegetables into your family.

Serves 16

Ingredients

275g carrots, peeled, thinly sliced, boiled for 15 minutes
     drained and mashed
Either 175g dairy-free **&/or** soya-free margarine
175g caster sugar
3 eggs, beaten
150g gluten-free flour
2 teaspoons baking powder
1 ½ teaspoons cinnamon
¼ teaspoon nutmeg

Method

1) Pre-heat the oven to 180C/375F/Gas Mark 5. Grease and flour a 25cm square cake tin.

2) Cream together the margarine and sugar. Add slowly, the mashed carrots and beaten eggs, mix well.

3) In a separate bowl, sift together the gluten-free flour, spices and baking powder. Then add this, one spoonful at a time to the carrot mixture and keep stirring until all the ingredients are combined and lump free. (Using an electric food mixer will help to achieve good results.)

4) Place the cake mixture into the cake tin and bake for 20 minutes in a pre-heated oven until the cake is brown, springy to touch and a cake skewer comes away clean when inserted. Leave to cool on a wire cooling rack before serving.

Toddler Chocolate Birthday Cake

A bit more sophisticated than the traditional sponge cake (if you prefer a sponge cake use the chocolate pudding recipe on page 74 but replace the muscovado sugar with castor sugar). The buckwheat flour gives the cake a pleasant nutty flavour which works well with the chocolate and cinnamon. Adding mashed potato ensures the cake stays remains moist. Undecorated, sliced and wrapped in foil portions, this cake freezes well.

Serves 16-20

Ingredients

Either 100g dairy-free **&/or** soya-free margarine
300g muscovado sugar
350g buckwheat flour
2 ¼ teaspoon gluten-free baking powder
200g mashed potato cooled*
200g 70% + plain dairy-free **&/or** soya-free chocolate, melted.
250ml cold water
2 teaspoon instant coffee dissolved in 1 tablespoon boiling water
1 teaspoon ground cinnamon
4 eggs, beaten

To decorate
glacé icing or melted plain chocolate and a selection of glacé cherries, dairy/wheat free small sweets or dragees,

(* If you do not have any ready-prepared mashed potato then bake a potato in the microwave, scoop out the cooked potato and mash with 1 tablespoon of water before cooling).

Method

1) Pre-heat your oven to 180C/375F/Gas Mark 5.

2) Grease and line with greaseproof paper, a 25cm square cake tin

3) Cream the margarine and sugar together.

4) Melt the chocolate over a pan of boiling water or in a bowl in the microwave for 1 minute. Once the chocolate is melted add the dissolved coffee. Then add the mashed potato. Beat the mixture thoroughly.

5) Add the chocolate mixture to the creamed margarine and sugar mixture. Then add the beaten eggs and mix well.

6) In a separate bowl sieve together the buckwheat flour, cinnamon and baking powder. Stir into the potato mixture.

7) Add the cold water and beat until the mixture is smooth.

8) Pour the cake mixture into the cake tin and cook for 25 minutes in the pre-heated oven. The cake will be springy to touch and a cake tester should come out clean when inserted.

9) Leave the cake to cool for ten minutes before turning out onto a wire cooling rack. Once the cake is completely cool decorate with melted chocolate or glacé icing and your choice of sweets or dried fruit.

8: Breakfasts

Apple and Cinnamon Muffins

Fruity muffins are ideal as a weekend breakfast treat but they can be enjoyed anytime and are a useful addition to lunch boxes. It is also easy to vary the fruit: try 50g of fresh blueberries or cranberries instead of the apple.

Makes 16

Ingredients

Either 250g plain flour
      or 125g buckwheat flour + 125g rice flour
1 teaspoon baking powder
Either 250ml milk
      or 250ml oat or rice or soya milk
2 eggs
175g dark brown soft sugar
Either 100g butter or margarine
      or 100g dairy-free **&/or** soya-free margarine
2 small cooking apples, peeled, cored and cubed
1 teaspoon ground cinnamon

Method

1) Pre-heat the oven to 180C/375F/Gas Mark 5. Place 16 muffin cases into a muffin tin.

2) Mix the flour, baking powder, cinnamon and apple cubes together in a bowl.

3) In a second bowl, melt the butter **or** margarine. (This takes approximately 40 seconds in the microwave.)

4) Add the sugar, eggs and milk to the melted fat and mix well. Fold the flour and apple mixture into melted ingredients.

5) Pour the mixture into the muffin cases taking care not to overfill them.

6) Bake for 15-20 minutes until they are well golden, risen and springy to touch. Then place on a wire rack to cool.

7) Enjoy freshly baked or freeze ready for another occasion.

Banana Smoothie

Vary the flavour of this basic Smoothie recipe as much as you like: try using strawberries, raspberries, mango, peach or a mixture of different soft fruits. Alternatively you can change the ice-cream – strawberry, raspberry ripple, chocolate, toffee and butterscotch all work well.

Ingredients

Either 250ml milk
       or 250 ml oat, rice or soya milk
2 bananas
Either 2 scoops of vanilla dairy ice-cream
       or 2 scoops dairy-free vanilla ice-cream
       (either oat or soya based)
       or home-made vanilla ice-cream (see p182)

Method

1 Place all the ingredients into an electric blender or smoothie maker. Blitz on full power for 1 minute.

2 Pour into a glass and drink straight away.

Bread

Dairy-free bread is easy to make since most basic bread recipes rely on oil and water for the liquid and do not need milk. Even if you want to make the dough richer by replacing all or some of the water with milk then either oat, rice or soya milk will work well.

Wheat-free bread is a different matter. The springy soft, moist bread that wheat produces is unique. Gluten-free flour produces drier bread that is harder, darker in colour, closer in texture and in many ways more like wholemeal bread.

However, the good news is that the nutritional content of gluten-free bread is excellent and since it has a pleasant flavour, once you are used to it, you won't need to feel hard done by when every one else gets out their sandwiches.

Gluten-free breads are best enjoyed fresh and hot. If there is any bread left on the day it is made then slice it, put pairs or individual slices into sandwich bags and freeze. You can just defrost or toast slices as needed. Re-heating the thawed bread definitely makes it taste better so you may want to microwave defrost rather than just leaving it out to thaw at room temperature.

Gluten-free loaves are becoming more readily available in supermarkets but they are not always dairy and/or soya-free and are also expensive. It really is worth buying your own bread-maker if you are making gluten-free bread. We have found that the results you get using a bread maker are better textured, more consistent and time saving, compared with those you can achieve with hand-baking.

Of course, other members of the family who can enjoy delicious home-baked wheat breads will be happy too!

Basic loaf

In our house the delicious scent of freshly baked bread and the 'Finished!' beep of the bread-maker have even the youngest members of the family toddling into the kitchen demanding 'Bread!' - only to discover the oldest have already started munching.

When you first make wheat-free bread be prepared for a different taste and a chewier texture. If you are able to tolerate buckwheat, then using it will make your loaf look denser - but its taste is much nearer to wheat bread.

Ingredients

These quantities make a ½ kilo loaf.

350ml water at hand hot temperature
2 tablespoon olive oil
Either 500g strong bread flour
      or 250g gluten-free bread flour + 250g buckwheat flour + 1 ½ teaspoon xanthan gum + 1 teaspoon baking powder
25g caster sugar
15g (or 1 sachet) dried easy-blend yeast*

* if you use tinned or dried yeast, or fresh yeast then blend the yeast and sugar together and work it to a smooth paste before adding to the water and oil.

Bread-maker method

1. Pour the water and oil into the bread pan.

2. Place the flour(s), xanthan gum, and baking powder on top of the liquid so that it is covered. Then sprinkle on the sugar and sachet of dried easy-blend yeast*.

3. Set your bread machine to its basic white bread programme, and (if it has this option) select the lightest crust option before turning the machine on.

4. Once the machine has completed its cycle turn the bread out onto a wire rack to cool.

Hand method

(This produces a heavier loaf than the bread-maker version)

1) Sift the flour(s) in a large mixing bowl. Add the other dry ingredients and mix well.

2) Make a well in the centre of the flour mixture and pour in the warm water. Mix until you have dough that holds together. Don't worry if the dough feels quite sticky.

3) Next, grease and flour an 800g loaf tin. Place the dough in the tin. Then cover the tin with cling film (or a wet plastic bag or damp tea towel). Leave the tin in a warm place for 40 minutes so that the yeast can work and make the dough rise.

If you are using strong wheat bread flour then your loaf will be much better, if, at this stage, you take it out of the tin to re-knead for a few minutes. Once you have knocked the dough back down to a smaller size place it back in the tin and allow rising once more. Do not knock back a gluten-free loaf.

4) Pre-heat oven to 200C/425F/Gas Mark 7

5) Place the risen dough into the pre-heated oven. (The temperature of the oven that the bread goes into is important, as it has to kill the yeast immediately.) Bake for 15-20 minutes until the loaf has a light, golden colour crust and sounds hollow when you tap its bottom.

6) Turn the cooked loaf out onto a wire rack and leave to cool. Eat fresh or slice and freeze in pairs.

Since wheat-free bread goes stale quicker than wheat bread, the Best Bread Use flow chart opposite will give you lots of ideas on how to make the best use of your loaf.

Best Bread Use

Age of bread	Best used for:
The day it is made	Sandwiches Cutting into slices, putting in a plastic bag and freezing.
1 day-old bread	Toast Pizza Base Bread and Butter pudding p172
2+ days old – when it has become drier	Eggy Breads p101 Fried Bread Bread Pudding p198 Apple Charlotte p166
2+ days old and dry	Make into bread crumbs and use for: Crunchy chicken p120 Crunchy pork p120 Fish bites p125 Meat balls p132 Smoked haddock fishcakes p158 Queen of puddings p190 Sultana and carrot puddings p192

Sausage, Beans and Potato Cakes

My Dad used to get up early to make sure we always faced school with a hearty cooked breakfast inside us. This combination was my favourite. Sadly I have never managed to produce a cooked breakfast on a school day but the same dish delights my children at tea time.

Serves 4

Ingredients

Either 4 meat sausages
>   **or** 4 wheat-free **&/or** dairy-free **&/or** soya-free sausages

200g gluten-free baked beans
400g mashed potato *[or 4 large baking potatoes cooked in the microwave, insides scooped out and mashed with butter or dairy-free and/or soya-free margarine]*
Either 4 tablespoons plain flour
>   **or** 4 tablespoons gluten-free flour

2 teaspoons gluten-free baking powder
Either 50g butter
>   **or** 50g dairy-free **&/or** soya-free margarine

2 tablespoons olive oil

Method

1) Cook the sausages under the grill according to manufacturer's instructions. Warm the beans in a saucepan over a low heat.

2) In a mixing bowl combine the flour and baking powder then rub in the margarine until the mixture resembles fine breadcrumbs.

3) Stir in the mashed potato. Then knead this dough till it leaves the sides of the bowl clean.

4) Shape the dough into cakes and cook in a hot, lightly oiled frying pan. Turn each cake over once so it browns on both sides.

5) On each plate, arrange a face: the potato cakes are giant eyes, the sausage is the nose and a large spoonful of baked beans is the mouth. (You can even add ketchup spikes of hair.) Serve hot.

Scotch Pancakes with Maple Syrup

We are real fans of maple syrup in our house and enjoy these with ice-cream as a pudding. However, these are just as delicious eaten warm from the pan spread with butter (or margarine) and jam as part of a high tea. Once cold these pancakes are a useful snack and a welcome treat in lunchboxes.

Serves 4-6

Ingredients

Either 100g plain flour
1 teaspoon baking powder
       or 50g buckwheat flour + 50g rice flour + ½ teaspoon bicarbonate of soda + 1 teaspoon cream of tartar*
25g caster sugar
1 egg beaten
Either 150 ml milk
or 150ml oat, rice or soya milk
50 ml sunflower oil
150ml maple syrup

* Instead of the mixture of bicarbonate of soda and cream of tartar it is possible to use 1 ½ teaspoons of gluten-free baking powder as the raising agent with the buckwheat flour but the results are not as good.

Method

1) Mix the flour, raising agent and sugar together. Make a well in the centre and pour in the beaten egg. Stir well.

2) Add half the milk and mix well. Then add the rest of the milk and beat until you have a thick batter the consistency of thick cream.

4) Place two tablespoons of olive oil in a heavy based frying pan and heat until hot. Reduce the heat from full to half-heat. Then place three separate spoonfuls of batter in the pan keeping them well apart. After 1-2 minutes turn the pancakes. Cook till golden brown on both sides.

3) Repeat step 3 until all the mixture is used up. Serve the pancakes hot, drizzled with maple syrup.

9: Lunchbox, picnic food and snacks

Butternut Squash and Sweet Potato Soup

A beautiful vibrant orange, this soup is warming, delicious and packed with vitamins. If you would like a spicier flavour then, when you are frying the onion, add all of the following:
1 teaspoon chilli powder,
1 teaspoon ground coriander,
1 teaspoon garam masala
1 teaspoon cumin.

Serves 4

Ingredients

2 tablespoon olive oil
1 onion, peeled and chopped
1 butternut Squash, peeled, seeded and chopped
1 large sweet potato, peeled and chopped
400ml water
salt and freshly ground pepper

Method

1) Heat the olive oil in a large saucepan and add the chopped onions. Cook for 3-4 minutes to soften.

2) Add the Butternut Squash and sweet potatoes and stir for a further 3-4 minutes.

3) Add the water, salt and freshly ground pepper. Bring to the boil, then reduce the heat to a simmer for 20 minutes until the vegetables are very soft.

4) Purée the mixture in a blender, food processor or use a hand-held blender until smooth. Pour into a clean saucepan and reheat stirring all the time. Check the seasoning and consistency adding a little more water if it is too thick.

5) Serve hot.

Mushroom Soup

Subtle and satisfying. This soup's flavour can be varied by using different mushrooms or replacing the water with chicken stock. Although potato is not a traditional ingredient in mushroom soup, it is included here not only to thicken the soup but to make the soup more calorific.

Serves 4-6

Ingredients

500g mushrooms, wiped, cleaned and sliced
a handful of dried Porcini mushrooms
1 onion, peeled and finely chopped
2 potatoes, finely chopped
2 tablespoon olive oil
1 tablespoon fresh flat leaf parsley, chopped
1 tablespoon fresh thyme leaves
1 litre water
salt and freshly ground black pepper

Method

1) Re-hydrate the Porcini mushrooms by covering them in boiling water and leaving to stand for 30 minutes.

2) In a large pan or wok, heat the olive oil and fry the onions for 5 minutes. Add the fresh mushrooms and cook for a further five minutes to soften the onion and until water starts to come out of the mushrooms. Add the re-hydrated drained Porcini mushrooms, potato, parsley and thyme and water.

3) Bring the mixture to the boil, then reduce the temperature and simmer for 20 minutes, until the potatoes are soft.

4) Either blend with a hand blender or pour into a food processor or blender and blend until smooth.

5) Serve hot with bread.

Spicy Courgette and Apricot Soup

This bright, spicy soup is wonderfully warming.
Make sure that the curry paste is gluten-free &/or dairy-free &/or soya-free and nut-free as you require. Garam masala works well as an alternative to curry paste.

Serves 4-6

Ingredients

1-2 tablespoons curry paste (or powder)
2 tablespoons olive oil
600g courgettes, washed and diced
200g dried, stoned apricots, chopped
800ml boiling water

Method

1 Place 2 tablespoons of olive oil in a saucepan, add and fry the curry paste for 1 minute. Quickly add the courgettes and cook for a further 2-3 minutes stirring all the time.

2 Add the apricots and boiling water. Bring to the boil and then simmer for 20 minutes until all the ingredients have softened.

3 Remove the pan from the heat and then use a hand blender, blender or food processor blend the mixture into a smooth thick soup. More boiling water can be added if you prefer a thinner soup.

4 Serve hot with fresh bread.

Tomato Soup

Who doesn't love tomato soup? Its cheerful colour, warmth and delicate flavour have made it a national favourite. This version is a satisfying meal in its own right and is another school, or office, lunchtime winner.

Serves 4-6

Ingredients

1 onion, peeled and chopped
1 carrot, peeled and chopped
2 sticks of celery, washed and chopped
2 potatoes, peeled and cubed
1 tablespoons fresh basil, chopped
4 slices of streaky bacon, chopped
1 x 400g tinned chopped tomatoes
1 tube tomato purée
salt and freshly ground pepper
Either 1.4 litre beef stock, hot
      or 1.4 litre gluten-free beef stock, hot

Method

1) Put all of the ingredients into a large saucepan. Bring to the boil, stir well, cover and simmer for about an hour until all the ingredients are soft. Cool slightly

2) Pour the soup into a food processor, blender or hand blender to purée the soup until it is smooth.

3) Serve hot with fresh bread.

Note: To make this soup a vegetarian dish, remove the bacon and change the beef stock to vegetable stock.

Winter Vegetable Soup

There is nothing more warming on a cold winter's day than a bowl of chunky vegetable soup. This makes a really satisfying lunch (and travels well in a vacuum flask for packed lunches). But it's even nicer when you can curl up in front of the fire in the evening and dunk chunks of home-made bread in it.

Serves 4-6

Ingredients

½ swede, peeled and diced
1 large potato, peeled and diced
1 carrot, peeled and cubed
1 parsnip, peeled and cubed
2 bay leaves
handful of chopped parsley
Either 1 litre vegetable stock, hot
        or 1 litre gluten-free vegetable stock, hot
salt and freshly ground pepper

Method

1) Place all the ingredients in a large saucepan. Bring to the boil and simmer for 20 minutes until all the vegetables are soft. Remove the bay leaves.

2) Either purée till it becomes a smooth soup using a hand held blender, or a food processor, or blender.

3) Serve hot with fresh bread.

Eggy Breads

Delicious for breakfast, lunch or tea. Serve hot with bacon, sausages, fried tomatoes, grilled mushrooms, etc., And just for the record, we think the gluten-free bread gives a better result than wheat bread.

Serves 4

Ingredients

Either 4 slices of wheat bread
      or 4 slices gluten-free **&/or** dairy-free **&/or** soya-free bread
2 eggs, beaten
bacon fat or olive oil for frying

Method

1) Cut the bread up into 4cm wide strips. Dip these in the beaten egg.

2) Have a hot frying pan ready. Then either add the olive oil or if you've just been frying bacon use the fat residue.

3) Cook the eggy breads for about 1 minute on each side until golden brown and the egg is set.

4) Serve hot.

Ham and Sweetcorn Fritters

Quick to make and a great way of hiding some of those '5 a day' fruit and vegetable portions in a tasty treat. Using gram flour (made from chickpeas) gives the fritters a faintly nutty flavour that combines really well with the basil and spices. You can easily vary the vegetable to use up any leftovers you have got in the fridge – try cooked potato, cooked peas, celery, red or green pepper, pepperoni or cooked meat.

Serves 4-6

Ingredients

Either 150 g plain flour
      or 150g *gram flour (chickpea flour)
½ teaspoon salt
2 eggs
Either 150ml milk
      or 150ml oat or rice or soya milk
a twist of freshly ground pepper
1 teaspoon ground cumin
1 teaspoon ground chilli powder
3 tablespoon fresh basil, finely chopped
50g tin sweetcorn
2 slices already-cooked ham, chopped.
2 spring onions, washed and chopped (use scissors)
3 tablespoon olive oil for frying

Anyone with an allergy to nuts should avoid gram flour because it is made from chick peas.

Method

1) Sieve the flour, salt, cumin, pepper and chilli powder into a mixing bowl.

2) Make a well in the middle, crack in the eggs, and beat well. Then pour in your choice of milk and beat until the batter is smooth.

3) Stir in the chopped basil, sweetcorn, ham and onions.

4) Heat the oil in a frying pan on a moderate heat for a few minutes. Once the oil is hot, spoon a tablespoon of mixture into the pan.

5) Cook each fritter for 1-2 minutes till the underside is crisp and golden, then flip over and cook the other side. Remove the cooked fritters from the pan and place them on a piece of kitchen paper on a plate. Pat them with another piece to get rid of any excess oil.

6) The fritters are great served with mixed salad leaves and mayonnaise, or baked beans.

For extra tang, teenagers (and adults) will love dipping fritters in 'Thai Sweet Chilli sauce' and they are also a handy addition for packed lunches and picnics.

Hot Dogs

Although hot dogs are a quick meal when made with bought bread rolls and sausages, with a little preparation the whole family can enjoy the same meal. If you make your own bread dough then adding a few teaspoons of fresh, chopped or dried herbs (e.g. basil rosemary, oregano or marjoram will make the rolls even tastier.

Serves 12

Ingredients

Either 12 wheat-bread finger rolls
      or 1 quantity of bread dough (follow
      the recipe on p86)
Either 12 x 100% meat sausages
      or 12 x dairy-free **&/or** wheat-free **&/or**
      soya-free sausages

Method

1) Turn the dough out onto a floured work top. Divide the dough into 12 pieces. With floured fingers, roll each piece into a finger roll shape and place on a greased and floured baking sheet. Cover the fingers with a wet plastic bag and leave to rise for 15-20 minutes until the dough springs back when you press it with a finger.

2) Pre-heat your oven to 200C/425F/Gas Mark 7. Bake the finger rolls in the centre of the pre-heated oven for 10-15 minutes until the roll sounds hollow when tapped. (The gluten free rolls will look very pale)

3) Prick the sausages and cook in the oven at the same time as the bread dough for 15-20 minutes until golden brown in colour and thoroughly cooked. (If you are using ready-made rolls pre-heat the oven to 200C/425F/Gas Mark 7 and cook the sausages, add the rolls when the sausages are almost cooked to warm them up.)

4) Slice open the rolls and place a sausage inside. Enjoy eating them plain or add fried onions, tomato ketchup, mustard or barbecue sauce.

Onion Bhajias

These are amazingly easy to make and delicous as a starter before eating curry or eaten as a snack or party food. Less authentic (but rather tasty) is the habit of dipping bhajias in tomato ketchup or sweet chilli sauce...

Makes 20

Ingredients

3 onions, peeled and thinly sliced
400g potato, grated
200g *gram flour
2 teaspoon ground cumin
1 teaspoon ground coriander
1 teaspoon turmeric powder
1 teaspoon mixed spice
½ teaspoon salt
olive oil for shallow frying

Anyone with an allergy to nuts should avoid gram flour because it is made from chick peas.

Method

1) Mix together the gram flour, spices and salt. Then add the sliced onions and grated potato and stir well (it is well worth using a food processor to grate and slice this quantity of vegetables).

2) Fill the frying pan to a 1cm depth with oil and heat the pan till the oil is hot. Place small spoonfuls of the mixture into the hot pan.

3) Keep turning the bhajias over in the hot oil until they are golden brown on all sides. (It is important to make sure that the mixture is thoroughly cooked – the raw mixture tastes awful!)

4) Once cooked, the Bhajias should be placed on a piece of kitchen paper on a plate to drain off the excess oil.

5) Serve hot.

Party Pizzas

This is fab finger food served hot or cold and your guests will thank you for offering them something that doesn't crumble all over their clothes. You can vary the toppings to suit your party and use different shaped cutters (stars, hearts, flowers…) to suit the mood. Of course, these are also great snacks for lunchboxes and as part of on-the-go lunches, or you can make use of the same recipe to make a large pizza base for a more substantial meal.

Makes 12

Ingredients

Either 100g self-raising flour
       or 100g gluten- free flour
       + 1 teaspoon gluten-free baking powder
Either 50g butter or margarine
       or 50g dairy-free **&/or** soya-free margarine
100g polenta
½ teaspoon salt
150ml cold water
½ tube of tomato purée
4 teaspoon dried mixed herbs
3 spring onions finely chopped (use scissors)
50g smoked bacon

Optional topping
Either 100g mozzarella, grated
       or 100g buffalo mozzarella

Method

1) Pre-heat the oven to 180C/375F/Gas Mark 5.

2) Grease and flour a baking sheet.

3) Place the flour, polenta, baking powder and salt in a bowl. Then rub in the butter or margarine using your finger tips until they resemble fine breadcrumbs. Make a well in the centre and stir in enough water to form a soft dough. (Alternatively, you can use a food processor)

4) Turn the dough out onto a floured work surface and knead lightly. Roll out to approximately 1.5 cm thick. Using a 6cm fluted round cutter, make about 12 rounds. Place them on the greased baking sheet.

5) Spread 1teaspoon of tomato purée on each round. (The back of a teaspoon is a good tool for doing this.) Then sprinkle with mixed herbs, and chopped spring onions.

6) If you are not using a cheese topping then cut the bacon into strips and use to cover the top of the pizza. If you are using the cheese topping, then chop the bacon finely and sprinkle over the pizza, then sprinkle with grated cheese or cut thin pieces of cheese to fit on to the top of each pizza.

7) Bake for 10-15 minutes until the pizza base is cooked and the cheese is golden in colour or cooked.

8) Serve hot or cold.

Savoury Tart

Savoury tarts are popular and versatile. Served hot or cold, with a salad or with potatoes and vegetables, they are a welcome sight at parties, tea-time, or next day in lunchboxes. Vary the filling to suit your family's taste e.g. mushroom and ham, smoked salmon and peas, roasted Mediterranean vegetables, tuna and sweetcorn...

Serves 6

Ingredients

Either 200g plain flour
       or 100g gluten free plain flour
       + 100g rice flour + pinch of salt
Either 100g butter cut into small pieces
       or 100g dairy-free **&/or** soya-free margarine
       cut into small pieces
1 egg beaten
2-3 tablespoon cold water
1 tablespoon olive oil
100g lean bacon, chopped
2 spring onions, finely chopped (use scissors)
2 large eggs, beaten
salt and freshly ground pepper
Either 150ml dairy or goat's milk
       or 150ml oat, rice or soya milk
Optional topping
Either 100g cheddar or sheep's cheese, grated
       or 100g soya cheese slices, chopped – *these may contain dairy products so check the list of ingredients carefully*

Method

1) Pre-heat the oven to 190C/400F/Gas Mark 6.

2) Place the flour (and salt if used) in a mixing bowl. Then rub the fat lightly into the flour using your fingertips until the mixture resembles fine breadcrumbs.

3) Add the beaten egg and water. Combine the mixture using a knife until it clings together forming a soft dough and leaves the sides of the bowl clean. Place the dough on a lightly floured work surface and knead lightly into a smooth round ball. (Refrigerate gluten free pastry for 15 minutes before beginning the next stage.)

4) Roll out the pastry and line a 20cm flan dish. (The gluten free pastry will be difficult to handle so try rolling it out on a board covered with cling film. Then lift the cling film and slide the pastry into the dish.)

5) Chill the flan case for 15 minutes before lining it with greaseproof paper or silver foil and adding baking beans to weigh it down. Bake the pastry case for 10 minutes. Remove the paper or foil and baking beans, then cook for 5 minutes until the pastry is dry but not brown.

6) Pour the olive oil into a frying pan and place over a moderate heat. Fry the bacon and spring onions until slightly brown. Place them in the prepared flan dish.

7) Beat together the eggs and your choice of milk and season well. Pour into the flan dish, then, if using, cover with your choice of grated or sliced cheese.

8) Reduce the oven temperature to 150C/325F/Gas Mark 3. Place the flan dish on a baking tray and cook for 30 minutes until the quiche is golden brown and the egg custard filling has set. Serve hot or cold.

Spanish Omelette (Tortilla)

Great when eaten cold on the beach in summer or as part of country picnics but just as good served piping hot on icy days - bringing the promise of happy holidays still to come.

Serves 4

Ingredients

6 eggs, beaten
400g potatoes peeled and thinly sliced
1 small red pepper, chopped into small pieces
50g mushrooms, wiped clean and thinly chopped
1 red onion, peeled and finely chopped
1 tablespoons fresh thyme, chopped
50g smoked ham, chopped
8 green, pitted, Spanish olives, sliced
9 tablespoons olive oil

Method

1) Heat 3 tablespoons olive oil in a frying pan which has a lid. When the oil is hot, add the potato slices and stir them to coat them in the olive oil. Put the lid on the pan and fry them over a low heat, until soft and cooked through. You will need to turn the potatoes frequently and shake the pan to help prevent them from sticking. When the potatoes are cooked remove them from the pan and set aside on a plate.

2) Add 3 tablespoons olive oil to the frying pan, and place it over a high heat. Fry the pepper, mushrooms and onion until soft and slightly brown.

3) In a large bowl place the beaten egg, cooked potatoes, fried vegetables, thyme, ham and seasoning. Mix thoroughly.

4) Return the pan to the heat and add the remaining olive oil. When the oil is hot, pour in the egg mixture and reduce the heat to a low setting. Cook the omelette for 20-25 minutes without stirring the mixture until there is no raw egg left on the surface.

5) Pre-heat the grill on a high setting. Then place the frying pan carefully under the grill for 2-3 minutes to brown off the top of the omelette.

6) Sprinkle the chopped olives over the omelette and serve cut into wedges.

10: Main Courses

Beef Casserole

Another week-day staple, this casserole is ideal served with new potatoes and a green vegetable.

Serves 4-6

Ingredients

900g braising steak, cubed
3 tablespoons olive oil
salt and freshly ground pepper
Either 3 tablespoons plain flour
      or 3 tablespoons gluten-free plain flour
1 large onion, peeled and diced
2 sticks celery, diced (optional)
3 carrots, cut into thin slices or stick
1 small swede, peeled and cubed, small
Leaves from 3 stems of fresh thyme
      (or 2 teaspoon dried thyme)
Either 300ml beef stock, hot
      or 300ml gluten-free beef stock, hot
2 tablespoon redcurrant jelly

Method

1) Pre-heat the oven to 180C/375F/Gas Mark 5.

2) Coat the diced beef in the seasoned flour.

3) Heat the oil in a large frying pan, and when hot fry the onions and celery until softened and slightly brown in colour. Add the meat and fry for a further 3-4 minutes turning it over until the meat is browned and sealed on all sides. Transfer to the casserole dish.

4) Add the carrots, swede, thyme and beef stock to the meat.

5) Place the lid on the casserole and cook for 1 ½ hours. (To slow down the cooking time, reduce the oven temperature to 150C/325F/Gas Mark 3 and cook for 3 hours.) Stir occasionally and add 3 tablespoons water if the sauce becomes too thick.

6) Just before serving add the redcurrant jelly and adjust the seasoning.

7) Serve hot.

Tip:
This dish can also be cooked in a slow cooker.

Chicken Casserole

A tasty weekday dinner that works well with boiled rice and green beans. If you like a richer tomato flavour, add a tube of tomato purée to the casserole in step 4.

Serves 4

Ingredients

4 chicken joints or breasts
6 tablespoon olive oil
Either 3 tablespoon plain flour
       or 3 tablespoon gluten-free plain flour
1 large onion, peeled and diced
2 sticks celery, sliced and thinly chopped (optional)
100g mushrooms, sliced
75g bacon, de-rinded and chopped
Either 300ml chicken stock, hot
       or 300ml gluten-free chicken stock, hot
1 X 400g tinned chopped tomatoes
3 tablespoon fresh basil, chopped
salt and freshly ground black pepper.

Method

1) Pre-heat the oven to 180C/375F/Gas Mark 5

2) Heat 3 tablespoons of olive oil in a frying pan, and add the onion, celery, mushrooms and bacon. Fry until softened and slightly brown. Remove from the frying pan and place in a large casserole dish.

3) Add another 3 tablespoons of olive oil to the frying pan. Meanwhile coat the chicken breasts in the seasoned flour and fry for 2-3 minutes turning so that all sides are sealed and the chicken is lightly browned. Place the cooked chicken in the casserole dish on top of the vegetables and bacon.

4) Pour over the stock and tinned tomatoes. Add the chopped basil and stir well.

5) Cook for about 1-1 ½ hours until the chicken is tender and thoroughly cooked. (Insert a skewer into the thickest part of the meat and any juices should be clear.)

6) Adjust the seasoning and, if the sauce is too thick add 2-3 tbsp of boiling water to thin it down.

7) Serve hot.

Tip
This dish can be cooked in a slow cooker.

Creamy Chicken

We think the oat cream version is especially good if you are cooking this dish dairy-free. It makes a lovely meal served with jacket potatoes or boiled rice and hot vegetables. If you want a slightly more unusual dish, add a tin of chopped apricots to the sauce in step 5.

Serves 4

Ingredients

4 chicken breasts, washed
2 teaspoon dried thyme
3 tablespoon olive oil
1 small leek, chopped small
100g mushrooms wiped clean and sliced
Either 50g butter or margarine
      or 50g dairy- &/or soya-free margarine
Either 40g plain flour
      or 40g gluten-free plain flour
Either 250 ml milk
      or 250ml oat, rice, or soya milk
Either 150ml double cream
      or 150ml oat cream or soya cream
salt and freshly ground pepper

Method

1) Pre-heat the oven to 180C/375F/Gas Mark 5

2) Place the chicken breasts into a baking dish, drizzle with the olive oil and sprinkle with the dried thyme. Cover and bake for 30-40 minutes until the chicken is thoroughly cooked – the meat must be white all the way through and the juices should run clear when a skewer is inserted into the thickest part of the chicken.

3) Slowly melt the butter **or** margarine in a saucepan. Add the leek and mushrooms, cook for 3-4 minutes until softened and slightly browned. Sprinkle over the flour and mix well.

4) Slowly add the milk and stir well over the heat. Bring the sauce to the boil and continue to stir until the sauce thickens. Remove from the heat.

5) Chop the chicken into bite sized pieces, add them to the sauce and stir well. Add the cream **or** oat cream **or** soya cream and stir well. Season to taste.

6) Serve hot.

Crunchy Chicken

Chicken nuggets are another childhood favourite and the good news is that not only does your allergic/intolerant child not have to miss out, but the rest of the family will enjoy the healthy, tasty version too. In fact every one in our family prefers the crunchy polenta coating.

Crunchy chicken can be served with potatoes (or chips) and vegetables, to make a main meal. Alternatively, it is great as party food served with a tomato, chilli or barbecue sauce dip. Any leftovers (and there are never many) can find their way into tomorrow's lunchbox.

Serves 4

Ingredients

2 chicken breasts
Either 1 egg, beaten
       *or 2 tablespoons cornflour + 1-2 teaspoons water, mixed to a thick paste
Either 50g bread crumbs
       or 50g gluten-free **&/or** soya-free bread crumbs
       or 50g polenta
olive oil for frying

*the alternative to egg is offered so that this dish can be prepared for members of the family who are allergic/intolerant of egg. However, the recipe works best with egg if everyone can eat them.

Method

1) Wash the chicken breasts and remove their skin. Then slice into chunks approximately 7cm x 3cm.

2) Place the breadcrumbs **or** polenta on to either a piece of kitchen paper or a plate.

3) Dip the chicken into your choice of either beaten egg or cornflour mixture. Then coat with the breadcrumbs or polenta.

4) Coat the bottom of the frying pan with olive oil and heat up the pan. When it is hot add the chicken and fry, turning once, until it is golden brown on both sides. Check that the chicken is thoroughly cooked. Then place on a piece of kitchen paper, on a plate, to drain off the excess oil.

Tip:
You can vary the coating by adding 1 teaspoon mixed herbs to the crumb/polenta mix or if your family like spicy flavours try 1 teaspoon dried chilli powder instead.

Sliced pork fillet can be used instead of chicken breasts in this recipe.

Dhansak

Don't be put off by the long list of ingredients – this is easy to make, extremely tasty and very healthy. Nor do you have to stick to the vegetables listed if there are others you prefer. Just keep the overall quantities the same.

Serves 4-6

Ingredients

2 tablespoon olive oil
1 onion peeled and finely chopped
2 garlic cloves, peeled and crushed (optional)
1 teaspoon ground ginger
1 teaspoon ground coriander
1 teaspoon ground chilli
1 teaspoon turmeric powder
1 teaspoon garam masala
2 teaspoon cumin
½ teaspoon salt
1x 400g tinned chopped tomatoes
1 small cauliflower, cut into florets
1 bag spinach, washed
410g cannelloni beans (tinned, ready cooked)
600 ml water
1 tablespoon fresh chopped coriander leaves

Method

1) Heat the oil in a large pan. Fry the onion, garlic, spices and salt for 3 minutes.

2) Add the tomatoes, cauliflower and water and mix well. Then add the washed spinach, bring the mixture to the boil. Cover and simmer for 20 minutes.

3) Add the cannelloni bean, bring to the boil, cover and simmer for a further 10 minutes.

4) Just before serving sprinkle with the fresh coriander.

5) Serve hot.

Herby Potato Wedges

These tasty potato wedges can be served for supper with grilled meat or fresh from the oven as an accompaniment to barbecued meats or hotdogs. They can also be enjoyed as a TV snack (especially if you dip them in ketchup, salsa or mayonnaise).

Serves 4-6

Ingredients

1kg baking potatoes
150ml olive oil
1 ½ tablespoon dried mixed herbs

Method

1) Wash the potatoes then chop them into wedge shapes. Rinse them again to remove the excess starch.

2) Pre-heat the oven to 200C/425F/Gas Mark 7.

3) Pour the olive oil into a baking tin and heat the tray in the oven for a few minutes. Add the potatoes to the hot oil and sprinkle with the mixed herbs.

4) Cook the potatoes for 45 minutes until they are golden brown, remembering to turn them over every 15 minutes so they colour evenly.

5) Serve hot.

Fish Bites

The non-allergic members of our family prefer the polenta coating to breadcrumbs so try it out on yours because producing one version that every one loves makes life so much easier.

Serves 4

Ingredients

2 large tails of fresh haddock, skinned and washed.
Either 1 egg, beaten
     or 2 tablespoons cornflour + 1-2 teaspoons mixed to a thick paste
Either 50g polenta
     or 100g gluten-free breadcrumbs
olive oil for frying

Method

1) Cut the fish into 7cm x 3cm pieces.

2) Place the polenta or breadcrumbs onto either a piece of kitchen paper or a plate. Dip the fish into your choice of beaten egg or cornflour mixture, then coat with your choice of breadcrumbs or polenta.

3) Place the frying pan on a high heat. Coat the bottom of the pan with oil. When the oil is hot add the fish and fry on both sides until golden brown.

4) Place onto a plate with a piece of kitchen paper, to drain off the oil.

5) Serve hot with tomato, brown or tartare sauce.

Sunset Haddock

This is a lovely sauce with any white fish, but especially delicious with haddock. Although this is a quick meal to make, read the recipe through twice before you start just to make sure you know the order in which you need to prepare the ingredients.

Serves 4

Ingredients

1 butternut squash
olive oil for drizzling
1 teaspoon dried parsley
Either 250ml double cream
      or 250ml oat cream or soya cream
Either 250ml fish or vegetable stock, hot
      or 250ml gluten-free fish or vegetable stock, hot
4 x 100 -150g pieces of fresh haddock
salt and freshly ground black pepper
Either 25g butter or margarine for frying
      or 25g dairy-free &/or soya-free margarine for frying
Either 50g breadcrumbs
      or 50g gluten-free breadcrumbs
4 rashers of smoked streaky bacon, chopped small

Method

1) Pre-heat the oven to 180C/375F/Gas Mark 5. Slice the butternut squash in half. Place in a baking tin, drizzle with olive oil. Cover with foil and bake until soft – this takes approximately 1 hour.

2) Scoop out the cooked butternut squash, add mix with the dried parsley and your choice of cream. Then pour through a fine sieve to produce a really smooth sauce. Place the sauce in a pan, season with salt and pepper, then slowly stir in the fish or vegetable stock and gently warm the sauce but do not allow it to simmer or boil.

3) Place the haddock fillet with the skin-side facing down in a frying pan and cook for about 2-5 minutes (depending on its thickness). Meanwhile pre-heat your grill.

4) Sprinkle the top side of the fish with your choice of breadcrumbs and place a knob of your choice of butter **or** margarine on top. Then place the fish, still in the frying pan, under the grill. Cook until the fish is cooked through and the breadcrumbs are golden.

5) Meanwhile, fry the small pieces of bacon until they are crispy and crunchy.

6) To serve: pour some warm sauce onto a plate, then position the fish on it with the bread-crumbed side facing up. Next scatter some of the bacon pieces on top.

7) Serve hot with rice or new potatoes.

Gnocchi

Gnocchi makes such a nice change from pasta, rice and potatoes. Gnocchi works well with bolognese sauce, or a casserole, and, if you can tolerate dairy then it makes a tasty meal served dotted with melted butter and sprinkled with grated cheese or Parmesan.

Children can enjoy helping to make gnocchi – they can shape the ovals or form any other shape they fancy.

Serves 4-6

Ingredients

500g baking potatoes, washed and scrubbed
Either 200g plain flour (+extra for kneading)
      or 200g gluten-free flour (+ extra for kneading)
2 eggs, beaten
salt and freshly ground pepper

Method

1) Prick the potatoes and cook in a microwave until soft (approximately 8-10 minutes). Cool and peel away the skins.

2) In a large bowl, mash the potatoes. Then add the flour and a pinch of salt and pepper. Mix well

3) Next, make a well in the middle of the mixture and pour in the beaten egg. Then mix to form a dough.

4) Turn the dough out onto a cold work surface and knead with your hands until smooth. Take pieces of dough and roll them into fat sausage shapes. Then cut off pieces of the dough about 3cm long and shape them into ovals. Press a fork down onto each oval to flatten them on each side.

5) Half-fill a large pan with boiling water and bring the water to the boil. Work with batches of the gnocchi – drop them into the pan of boiling water and let them cook until they rise to the surface (this takes approximately 1-3 minutes.) Once they have risen to the surface allow them a further 20 seconds before scooping them out with a slotted spoon.

6) Serve hot.

Gluten-Free Pasta

If you don't have a pasta machine then it is still easy to roll the pasta out and cut it into large rectangles to use for lasagne or thin strips for tagliatelle.

Serves 4-6

Ingredients

150g *gram flour
½ teaspoon salt
2 large eggs, beaten
1 tablespoon olive oil

*Anyone with an allergy to nuts should avoid gram flour because it is made from chick peas.

Method

1) Place the gram flour and salt in a bowl. Make a well in the centre of the flour and pour in the beaten eggs and olive oil. Mix well with a fork, bringing the ingredients together to form a ball of dough.

2) Roll the dough out thinly or pass it through a pasta making machine.(Results are better when you use a machine.) Cut into shapes.

3) Lay your pasta on a floured surface and leave to dry.

4) To cook, bring a large pan of salted water to boil, and pour in a dash of olive oil. Add the pasta and cook for 8-10 minutes until it is *al dente* (soft but still has a bite).

5) Serve with the sauce of your choice.

Lime and Thyme Roast Chicken Joints

Bound to become a family favourite because not only is it delicious but it is easy to cook too. The recipe works just as well with lemon instead of lime, and using a whole chicken instead of pieces.

Serves 4

Ingredients

4 chicken joints
2 red onions, peeled and sliced
10g fresh thyme sprigs
2 limes, juiced
salt and freshly ground pepper
2 tablespoons olive oil for roasting

Method

1) Wash the chicken joints thoroughly, pat dry with kitchen paper and place them in a roasting dish.

2) Mix together the olive oil, lime juice, fresh thyme and seasoning and then pour over the chicken. Cover and marinate for at least 20 minutes (preferably longer - overnight in the fridge works well.)

3) Pre-heat the oven to 180C/375F/Gas Mark 5. Place the sliced onion over the chicken and cook in the pre-heated oven for 20 minutes. Then turn over the chicken and cook for a further 25 minutes. The chicken is done when it's golden in colour and when you pierce the thickest part of the joint with a skewer the juices are clear.

4) 4 Serve hot or cold.

Meatballs

Ideal for when friends come to tea. This quantity of meatball mixture will make approximately 12 meatballs. Uncooked meatballs freeze beautifully, ready for a busier day when you can serve them with wheat-free pasta and a vegetable sauce. Cooked leftover meatballs can be used next day in packed lunches.

Serves 4-6

Ingredients

Either 125g wholemeal breadcrumbs
       or 125g gluten-free breadcrumbs
       or 100g oats* + 2 tablespoons water
1 onion, finely chopped
1 tablespoons fresh flat parsley, finely chopped
1 tablespoons fresh basil, finely chopped
pinch of salt and pepper
400g lean minced beef
1 tablespoons red wine vinegar
1 egg, beaten
olive oil for cooking

(If your child has to avoid wheat or barley etc. then make sure the oats you buy are completely pure and not contaminated with other cerals.)

Method:

1) Pre-heat the oven to 180C/375F/Gas Mark 5.

2) First put the breadcrumbs (or oats and water), onion, parsley, basil, salt, pepper, minced meat and red wine vinegar in a large bowl and mix thoroughly. Then add the beaten egg and mix everything thoroughly once more.

3) Drizzle olive oil onto a baking tin. Then, taking small handfuls of the mince mixture, roll them into balls and place them on the baking tin.

4) Cook the meatballs for 10-15 minutes until they are golden brown.

5) Serve hot or cold with mashed potato and baked beans. (Check the baked beans are gluten-free if you need to avoid gluten).

Moroccan Ratatouille

Packed with vitamin-rich vegetables this fragrant dish is a really useful addition to your range of every-day dishes. Depending on which ingredients your family can tolerate it can be served with rice, quinoa, wheat or barley couscous and is easily turned into a full meal by adding chick peas or serving with meat.
If your family like their food hot and spicy then add a chopped chilli to the pan as you fry the onion.

Serves 4-6

Ingredients

2 tablespoon olive oil
1 large onion, peeled and chopped
1 stick of celery, washed and chopped
1 yellow pepper, washed and chopped
1 clove of garlic, peeled and crushed (optional)
1 parsnip, peeled and chopped into cubes
3 sweet potatoes, peeled and chopped into cubes
1 aubergine, washed, trimmed, chopped into cubes
300 ml boiling water
2 x 400g tins chopped tomatoes
125g dried, soft apricots, chopped
1teaspoon ground cinnamon
1 teaspoon turmeric
1 teaspoon ground coriander
salt and freshly ground pepper

Method

1) In a large frying pan or wok, heat the olive oil over a moderate heat and gently cook the onion, celery and garlic for 4-5 minutes until soft. Then stir in the cinnamon, coriander and turmeric.

2) Next stir in the aubergine and yellow pepper and cook for a further five minutes till they are softened.

3) Add the parsnip, sweet potato, apricots and tinned tomatoes. Season well with salt and pepper. Stir well. Add the boiling water and stir again. Bring to the boil, then reduce the heat to simmer the vegetables for 20-30 minutes until they are soft.

4) If the ratatouille needs thickening: leave the lid off the pan and simmer for a further 10-15 minutes to reduce the liquid. Keep stirring while you do this to ensure the right consistency and to make sure the vegetables do not catch and burn. Season to taste.

5) Serve hot in the winter and cold in the summer.

Moussaka

Using potatoes instead of aubergines makes this tasty dish more appealing to children (and gives them extra energy) but if your family enjoy them you can use the same quantity of aubergines washed and sliced in place of the potatoes.

If your family are able to tolerate sheep's yoghurt and cheese as an alternative to dairy then this is a particularly delicious combination.

Serves 4-6

Ingredients

700g potatoes, sliced
500g minced lamb
1 medium onion, peeled and finely chopped
2 tablespoons olive oil
1 x 400g tinned chopped tomatoes
2 bay leaves*
1 tablespoon fresh thyme, chopped*
1 tablespoon fresh mint, chopped*
salt and freshly ground pepper
2 eggs, beaten
Either 500g natural yoghurt
  or 500ml oat cream +1 teaspoon Dijon mustard
  or 500g natural soya yoghurt
1 teaspoon cornflour

Optional topping
Either 50g cheddar cheese, grated
  or 50g sheep pecorina romano

* dried herbs can be used but the result is not as good

Method

1) Boil the sliced potatoes for 5-8 minutes until soft. Then strain off the water.

2) Heat 1 tablespoon olive oil in a large frying pan. Fry the chopped onion for approximately 5 minutes until it is softened and beginning to turn golden brown.

3) Pre-heat the oven to 180C/325F/Gas Mark5.

4) Add the minced lamb and fry for 5 minutes on a high heat. Keep stirring the lamb to break up the mince and to ensure that all of it is browned. Pour off the excess fat from the lamb.

5) Add the tinned tomatoes, rinse the tin out with 100ml of water and add this to the meat. Add the bay leaf, mint thyme and seasoning and simmer for 15 minutes.

6) Grease a deep oven-proof dish. Cover the bottom with a layer of potatoes, then pour over some of the meat sauce. Continue with another layer of potatoes, then meat sauce etc. Finish with a layer of potatoes.

7) Beat together the eggs, yoghurt or oat cream and cornflour, season and pour over the top layer of potato slices. If you are using the topping ingredients sprinkle the top with cheese.

8) 8 Cook for 35-45 minutes until golden brown on top. Serve hot.

Paella

A brilliant way to use up leftovers, this dish is quick and versatile. You can make it with just vegetables or change the meat to fish or another type of meat to suit what you have in the fridge. You can make it with other types of rice but paella rice is really the best!

Serves 4-6

Ingredients

400g paella rice
Either 25g butter
        or 25g dairy-free **&/or** soya-free margarine
1 tablespoon olive oil
1 red onion, peeled and chopped small
1 red pepper, chopped small
½ teaspoon turmeric
1 clove garlic, crushed (optional)
25g frozen peas*
75g smoked ham, cubed
100g cooked chicken
Either 900ml chicken stock, hot
        or 900ml gluten-free chicken stock, hot

*** some people with nut allergies are also unable to tolerate peas. In that case use the same quantity of frozen sweetcorn if this can be tolerated.**

Method

1) In a wok or large frying pan, melt the butter or margarine and add the olive oil.

2) Fry the onion and pepper for 3-4 minutes to soften. Add the turmeric and crushed garlic and fry for 1 minute.

3) Stir in the paella rice, making sure each grain is coated in the oil mixture.

4) Pour the hot stock over the rice. Then stirring all the time, bring the mixture to the boil.

5) Reduce the heat to a low setting and simmer for 10 minutes.

6) Stir well then add the frozen peas, cooked chicken and ham. Gently simmer for a further 10 minutes stirring occasionally to prevent the rice from sticking.

7) Test the rice to check that it is soft, then serve hot.

Pork Casserole

This is delicious served hot with rice and green beans or new potatoes and carrots. It is sure to become a family favourite.

Serves 4-6

Ingredients

900g pork tenderloin, sliced
1 ½ onions, peeled and sliced
1 courgette, sliced
1 tablespoon white wine vinegar
6 tablespoon olive oil.
Either 3 tablespoon plain flour
      or 3 tablespoon gluten-free plain flour
Either 300 ml chicken stock, hot
      or 300 ml gluten-free chicken stock, hot
Either 150 ml milk
      or 150ml oat, rice or soya milk
2 teaspoon dried sage
2 teaspoon dried mustard or Dijon mustard
salt and freshly ground black pepper

Method

1) Pre-heat the oven to 180C/375F/Gas Mark 5.

2) Heat 3 tablespoons olive oil in a large frying pan over a medium heat. When the pan is hot add the onions and courgettes and fry until they are soft and slightly browned. Remove them from the pan and place in a large casserole dish.

3) Pour another 3 tablespoons of olive oil into the same pan and put it back over the heat. When the oil is hot add the pork slices and sprinkle them with the dried sage. Fry for 3-4 minutes until they are browned, then sprinkle the flour over the meat and continue to cook turning the meat over so that it gets coated in the flour and the flour is cooked. Place the meat in the casserole dish.

4) Slowly mix the hot stock and wine vinegar into the casserole. Stir in the mustard. Then pour in the milk and stir again. Season with salt and pepper.

5) Cover the casserole and cook in the oven for 1 ½ hours stirring occasionally and, if the sauce becomes too thick, add 2-3 tablespoons of water. (If you want the casserole to cook more slowly reduce the oven temperature to 150C/325F/Gas Mark 3 and cook for 3 hours).

Tip: This recipe can be cooked in a slow cooker.

Pork with Apricot Sauce

Not only is the apricot sauce a beautiful colour but it smells and tastes lovely. If you prefer you can use pork chops instead of the pork fillet or to ring the changes this sauce works beautifully with chicken breasts.

Serves 4-6

Ingredients

450g pork fillet
2 tablespoon olive oil
1 teaspoon dried sage or 1 tablespoon fresh sage, chopped
salt and freshly ground pepper

Sauce ingredients
1 medium sized onion, peeled and chopped
1 tablespoon olive oil
½ teaspoon dried thyme or 1 tablespoon fresh thyme, chopped
250g tinned apricots in juice
½ teaspoon cinnamon
Either 250ml chicken stock, hot
       or 250ml chicken stock, hot

Method

1) Pre-heat the oven to 180C/375F/Gas Mark 5.

2) Place the fillet on a baking tray and drizzle with 1 tablespoon of olive oil. Sprinkle with sage and seasoning then roast for 25-30 minutes until the pork is thoroughly cooked and none of the meat looks pink.

3) Heat 1 tablespoon of olive oil in a frying pan and add the onion and thyme. Cook for a few minutes until the onion is soft.

4) Add the apricots, cinnamon and chicken stock. Simmer, uncovered, for about 5 minutes so that the liquid reduces. Then blend the sauce to a smooth consistency (using a food processor, blender or hand held blender).

5) Slice the meat and pour the hot sauce over it. Serve hot.

Roast Pork with Sage

Another great meal for families with allergies or food intolerance as its naturally wheat, dairy and soya free!

Serves 4-6

Ingredients

Pork joint
2 teaspoons dried sage
2 tablespoons olive oil
salt

Method

1 Pre-heat the oven to 180C/375F/Gas Mark 5

2 Rinse the pork joint with cold water to clean and freshen the meat. Pat dry with kitchen paper. Then place in a roasting tin and score the pork rind with a sharp knife (if it hasn't already been done). Rub the dried sage into the score lines, then rub again with the oil and finally sprinkle generously with salt so that the crackling will be really crunchy.

3 Roast the pork in the oven for 15 minutes per 450g +15 minutes until the pork is tender.

4 Remove the crackling before serving and keep warm (but do not cover or it will soften.)

5 Carve the meat and serve hot with crackling, potatoes, vegetables, gravy (see p152) and apple sauce.

Roast Beef

Traditional and rich in iron, roast beef with all the trimmings is a winner (especially as no one has to miss out on Yorkshire Puddings - see the recipe on p146.)

Serves 4-6

Ingredients

1 joint topside beef
4 tablespoons olive oil or beef dripping
seasoning

Method

1) Pre-heat the oven to 190C/400F/Gas Mark 6

2) Place the olive oil/beef dripping in a roasting tin and put it in the oven to heat up.

3) Rinse the beef joint with cold water then pat dry with kitchen paper. Once the fat in the roasting tin is hot add the beef and season well. Cook for 20 minutes to brown and seal the meat.

4) Reduce the oven temperature to 170C /350F/Gas Mark 4 and cook to your taste for the time shown below:
    Rare – 20 minutes per 450g +20 minutes
    Medium – 25 minutes per 450g +25 minutes
    Well done – 30 minutes per 450g +30 minutes.

5) Once cooked, remove the meat from the roasting tin and stand it on a plate. Cover it with foil and allow to relax for 10 minutes before carving. Serve hot or cold.

Yorkshire Pudding

Okay, hands up! The wheat-free and dairy-free versions of these are a bit more spongy than the traditional wheat versions (It's the extra egg and baking powder that does it). But these ' G.F. Yorkies' are so loved by our family that on the rare occasion when any are left over after the main course they find their way into the pudding bowls with warmed golden syrup drizzled over them.

Serves 4-6

Ingredients

Either 125g plain flour + pinch of salt
       or 100g rice flour
       + 1 x 5ml teaspoon gluten-free baking powder
2 eggs, beaten
Either 300 ml milk
       or 300ml oat, rice or soya milk
3 tablespoons olive oil.

Method

1) Pre-heat the oven to 200C/425F/Gas Mark 7. Drizzle the oil into the bottom of each well in a muffin tin.

2) Mix the flour and salt or rice flour and baking powder in a bowl. Make a well in the centre and pour in the beaten eggs.

3) Add half the milk and stir into the flour using a spoon. Add the rest of the milk and beat the mixture until smooth. (An electric mixer is good to use at this stage.)

4) Place the muffin tin at the top of the hot oven for a few minutes until the oil is so hot that a slight haze can be seen. Then remove the tin, pour the batter into the muffin wells and pop the tin back into the oven.

5) Cook for 10-15 minutes until the puddings are well risen and golden brown.

6) Serve hot.

Roast Chicken

The marvellous thing about roast chicken is that it's always popular with children and you can keep the grown-ups interested by varying the herbs: marjoram, tarragon, basil, oregano, thyme, garlic...

Serves 4-6

Ingredients

1.4kg chicken (<u>thoroughly</u> thawed if it has been frozen)
4 tablespoons olive oil
2 tablespoons fresh flat parsley, chopped (or 2 teaspoons of dried)
2 tablespoons white wine vinegar
salt and freshly ground pepper

Method

1) Pre-heat the oven 180C/375F/Gas Mark 5.

2) Wash the chicken inside and out. Pat dry with kitchen paper. Then place in a roasting tin. Drizzle it with oil and wine vinegar before sprinkling on the parsley and seasoning well.

3) Reduce the oven temperature to 170C/350F/Gas Mark 4. Roast the chicken for 20 minutes per 450g plus 20 minutes. Turn the chicken over every 20 minutes.

4) To check the chicken is cooked pierce the thickest part of the chicken with a skewer. As you remove the skewer the juices should run out and be clear. If you see any blood the chicken is not yet cooked and should be returned to the hot oven to cook for a further 10 minutes before you check it again. Continue cooking for further ten-minute periods and checking until the meat is thoroughly cooked.

5) Serve with roast potatoes, root and green vegetables, gravy (see p152) and apple sauce.

Roast Leg of Lamb

The fragrance of rosemary and roast lamb filling the house on a Sunday always makes me feel like such a good mum. Lamb is such a useful meat in families with allergies because rarely are children allergic to it and it is easier to chew than beef.

Serves 4-6

Ingredients

1 leg of lamb
2 tablespoon olive oil
2 tablespoon red wine vinegar
10 fresh rosemary sprigs
salt and freshly ground pepper

Method

1) Pre-heat the oven to 190C/400F/Gas Mark 6.

2) Rinse the leg of lamb under the cold tap to clean and freshen the meat. Pat dry with kitchen paper. Then place it in a roasting pan.

3) Mix together the oil and red wine vinegar and brush over the lamb. Then make 10 slits in the skin of the lamb and insert the rosemary sprigs. Season with salt and pepper.

4) Cook for 20 minutes uncovered then cover the meat with foil and reduce the oven temperature to 170C/350F/Gas Mark 4 and cook to your taste using the following timings:
     medium – 25 minutes per 450g + 25 minutes
     well done – 30 minutes per 450g + 30 minutes.

5) Once cooked, remove the meat from the roasting tin and stand it on a plate. Cover with foil and allow to relax for 10 minutes before carving. Serve hot.

Gravy

Well, it wouldn't be roast dinner without gravy would it?

Serves 4-6

Ingredients

Either 4 tablespoon plain flour
     or 4 tablespoon gluten-free flour
Either 400ml stock
     or 400ml gluten-free **&/or** soya-free stock
     or 400ml water vegetables have been cooked in
1 tablespoon redcurrant jelly
1 teaspoon gravy browning

Method

1) Remove the cooked roast meat from the roasting tin.

2) Skim off and remove all but 2 tablespoons of the fat. Stir in your choice of flour and mix in any browned crumbs of meat left in the tin.

3) Slowly add the stock/vegetable water and keep stirring while you bring it to the boil. Then reduce the heat so that the gravy simmers. Add the gravy browning to darken the colour of the gravy.

4) Once the gravy is as thick as you want it to be season with salt and pepper and add the redcurrant jelly.

5) Pour into your gravy jug and serve with your hot roast dinner.

Tuna Pasta

The ingredients for this are usually in the store cupboard, making this a good spur-of-the moment family favourite.

Serves 4

Ingredients

1 onion, peeled and chopped
2 tablespoons olive oil
1 x 400g tinned chopped tomatoes
2 x 170g tinned tuna, drained and flaked
1 tube tomato purée
Either 1 handful fresh basil leaves chopped
      or 1tablespoons dried mixed herbs.
Either: 175g penne pasta
      or 175g wheat-free **&/or** soya-free pasta
1 teaspoon olive oil
1 bag ready salted crisps, crushed (optional)

Method

1) Boil the penne pasta in salted water with 1 teaspoon olive oil, until it still has a bit of a bite (*al dente*). Stir occasionally while cooking to stop the pasta sticking.

2) In a large frying pan or wok, heat the olive oil and fry the onion till soft. Add the tinned tomatoes and herbs. Stir well. Add the tuna and tomato purée mix well and bring to the boil. Then simmer for 5 minutes.

3) Add the cooked, drained pasta to the tuna sauce and mix well.

4) Serve the tuna pasta hot, with sprinkled crisps on top.

Shepherd's Pie

A mid-week dish that can be made up to 24 hours in advance, then refrigerated and cooked when everybody comes in tired and hungry at the end of the day. Although this recipe is for beef mince it will taste just as delicious if you use either lamb or turkey mince instead.

Serves 4-6

Ingredients

3 tablespoons olive oil
1 small onion, peeled and finely chopped
1 medium leek, finely chopped
1 large carrot, peeled and diced small
100g mushrooms, wiped clean and diced small
250g lean minced beef
2 tablespoon red wine vinegar
Either 300ml beef stock, hot
       or 300ml gluten-free **&/or** soya-free stock, hot
8 fresh basil leaves, chopped
2 teaspoons dried mixed herbs
1x 400g tinned chopped tomatoes
1 tube of tomato purée
salt and freshly ground pepper
600g floury potatoes, peeled, cut into 5cm chunks
Either 25g butter + splash of milk
       or 25g dairy-free **&/or** soya-free margarine
       + splash of oat, rice or soya milk

Method

1) Place the olive oil in a large frying pan or wok. Heat the pan and then add the onion, leek and carrot. Fry them on a high heat for approximately 5 minutes until the vegetables are starting to soften. Stir in the minced beef and red wine vinegar and, still stirring, cook until the beef is lightly browned.

2) Stir the hot stock into the meat. Then add the chopped basil leaves, mixed herbs, tinned tomatoes, mushrooms and seasoning. Stir thoroughly once more then cover and simmer for 30 minutes.

3) Pre-heat the oven to 180C/375F/Gas Mark 5.

4) Place the potatoes in a large pan of cold water and bring to the boil. Simmer for 15-20 minutes until soft and ready to mash. Drain the potatoes thoroughly then mash with your choice of butter or margarine and splash of milk. Season and set aside.

5) Stir the tomato purée into the mince. Then pour the meat mixture into a large, deep ovenproof dish. Pile the mashed potato on top and use a fork to spread it to the edges of the dish.

6) Cook the shepherd's pie for 30 minutes in the oven, until it is piping hot and just starting to brown on top. Serve with baked beans or vegetables.

(Note: **Make sure the baked beans are gluten-free if you are a Coeliac)**

Sweet Potato and Courgette Sauce

This is a very healthy and tasty sauce to pour over pasta and if you stir in ready cooked meat can become a more substantial meal. Thinned down with a little more stock this sauce becomes a delicious soup.

Serves 4

Ingredients

2 tablespoons olive oil
1 onion, peeled and diced
1 green pepper, diced
1 large sweet potato, peeled and diced
1 x 400g tin chopped tomatoes
1 large courgette, diced
1 teaspoon dried mixed herbs
Either 250ml vegetable stock, hot
      or 250ml gluten-free **&/or** soya-free vegetable stock, hot

Method

1) Heat the olive oil in large frying pan over a moderate heat. Then add the chopped onion and pepper and fry for 3-4 minutes to soften.

2) Add the sweet potato, courgette and fry for a further 5 minutes stirring from time to time.

3) Add the tin of tomatoes, vegetable stock and herbs and stir thoroughly. Bring to the boil. Then simmer for 25 minutes until the vegetables are softened.

4) Remove from the heat and allow to cool slightly before blending to desired consistency.

5) Serve hot with pasta, rice, cooked meat or just on its own. It is also good served cold with cold meat.

Smoked Haddock Fishcakes

We all know we should be feeding our children more fish because it is good brain food, and this is a delicious way to do it. You can vary the recipe by changing the fish to salmon (rich in omega 3) or tuna, which some children prefer.
Bite-size fish cakes are ideal as party food.

Serves 4-6

Ingredients

225g smoked haddock
450g potatoes, peeled and cubed into small pieces
Either 25g butter
        or 25g dairy-free **&/or** soya-free margarine
1 tablespoon fresh flat leaf parsley, chopped
½ tablespoon fresh coriander, chopped
50g sweetcorn
2 spring onions, chopped (use scissors)
salt and freshly ground pepper
2 eggs, beaten
Either 25g plain flour
+ 50g wheat breadcrumbs
        or 25g gluten-free flour
        +50g gluten-free **&/or** soya-free breadcrumbs
olive oil for frying

Method

1) Place the smoked haddock in a saucepan and cover with cold water. Bring to the boil and cook for 10 minutes. Drain away the water.

2) Boil the potatoes for 10 minutes in salted water. Then drain and mash them with your choice of butter or margarine.

3) Mix together the fish, mashed potato, parsley, coriander, sweetcorn, spring onions and seasoning. Add a little of the beaten egg to bind the mixture together.

4) On a lightly floured surface, shape the mixture into a roll. Slice it into 8 pieces and form these into cakes.

5) Coat each cake with beaten egg and then cover in your choice of breadcrumbs and flour.

6) Heat the olive oil in a frying pan and once it is hot fry the fishcakes until they are golden brown and crisp.

7) Place the cooked fishcakes on a piece of kitchen towel and pat with another piece to remove the excess fat.

8) Serve hot with salad, vegetables or baked beans. **(Use gluten-free baked beans if you are a Coeliac.)**

Spaghetti Carbonara

Quick to make, this becomes a very sociable tea when the children have the fun of serving themselves and building their pile of ingredients. (Who knows? The fun may continue as they reward your efforts by helping to wash up the pans and dishes afterwards.)

Serves 4

Ingredients

Either 225g spaghetti
       or 225g gluten-free spaghetti
275g smoked back bacon, cut into small pieces
½ leek, finely chopped
Either 250g double cream
       or 250g oat cream or soya natural yoghurt or soya
       cream
1 teaspoon cornflour
2 eggs
4 sprigs fresh thyme
salt and freshly ground pepper
100g mushrooms, wiped clean and finely chopped
½ red pepper, finely chopped
4 tablespoons olive oil

Optional:
Either grated parmesan cheese
       or dairy-free parmesan

Method

1) Cook the spaghetti: fill a large saucepan with hot water and add ¼ teaspoon salt and a splash of olive oil. Bring the water to simmering point and add the pasta. Stir well once, then bring it up to the boil and cook for 8-10 minutes until the texture is *al dente* (i.e. still has a bit of a bite – not too soft). Then drain well.

2) Meanwhile, place 2 tablespoons olive oil in a frying pan. Add the bacon and leek and fry until the bacon is golden in colour. Season and add the thyme to the pan.

3) Place the cream or yoghurt in a bowl. Add the two eggs and cornflour and beat well. Pour this mixture over the leek and bacon and cook gently over a low heat until the sauce thickens.

4) In a separate frying pan, pour in 2 tablespoons olive oil and then fry the mushrooms and red pepper together until the mushrooms are golden.

5) To serve: In a clockwise circle, put out separate bowls of spaghetti, carbonara sauce, mushroom and pepper mix, and the grated cheese. Each person takes it in turn to go round the circle of bowls (starting with the pasta) building a pile of their chosen ingredients.

Turkish Lamb

This lightly spiced, succulent lamb and apricot dish is sure to become a family favourite, as it is so easy to prepare. Ready for busy days, the dish can be made in advance and then frozen. When re-heating, bring it to the boil and simmer for 10-15 minutes to bring out the flavours.

Serves 4-6

Ingredients

2 tablespoons olive oil
1 onion, peeled and chopped
1 green pepper, washed and diced
1 aubergine, washed and diced
1 garlic clove, chopped
1 teaspoon cinnamon
3 whole cloves
400g lean, ready-diced lamb
1 x 400g tinned chopped tomatoes
100g ready-to-eat dried apricots, chopped
1 x 100g tin *chick peas, drained
1 teaspoon honey
salt and freshly ground pepper
Either 300ml vegetable stock, hot
        or 300ml gluten-free vegetable stock, hot
1 tube tomato purée

Anyone with an allergy to nuts should avoid chick peas. This recipe will still taste really delicious even if you omit this ingredient.

Method

1) Pre-heat oven to 190C/400F/Gas Mark 6.

2) Heat the oil in a large frying pan, and add the chopped onion, green pepper and garlic. Cook slowly until the vegetables are soft, but not browned.

3) Stir in the cinnamon and whole cloves and fry for 1 minute. Add the lamb. Cook these ingredients for a further 5 minutes, taking care to turn the lamb to make sure it is sealed.

4) Transfer the ingredients into a large (5 litre) oven-proof casserole dish. Then add the chopped tomatoes, aubergine, hot stock, apricots, seasoning, chick-peas and honey.

5) Put the covered casserole dish in the pre-heated oven for 20 minutes. Then check that the liquid has come to the boil before reducing the oven temperature to 150C/325F/Gas Mark 3. Cook for a further 1 ¼ - 1 ½ hours until the lamb is tender (or cook all day in a slow cooker).

6) Take the casserole out of the oven and stir in the tomato purée to thicken the sauce (or just add to the casserole if using the slow cooker). Taste the sauce and check the seasoning. Then return the casserole to the oven for a further ten minutes.

7) Serve with boiled rice or wheat-eaters can enjoy it with couscous. For a more unusual option (but not one to give people avoiding gluten) try serving this dish with boiled barley, or barley couscous.

11: Puddings

Apple Crumble

Delicious placed over other fruits, crumble topping cooks really well in the microwave making it a truly fast pudding – especially if you keep a container of crumble topping in the freezer, along with some frozen fruit. To make a single portion of crumble put a layer of frozen or fresh fruit in a ramekin dish, cover it with 3-4 tablespoons of topping mixture and cook for 2 minutes in the microwave.

Crumble that has been cooked in the microwave is quite moist but you will get a drier, crunchy texture if you bake it in the oven.

Serves 6

Ingredients

Fruit filling
700g cooking apples, peeled, cored and cubed
1 teaspoon mixed spice
50g caster sugar.

Topping
Either 75g butter or margarine
        or 75g dairy-free **&/or** soya-free margarine
Either 100g plain flour
        or 100g gluten-free flour
100g porridge oats*
Either 100g butter or margarine
        or 100g dairy **&/or** soya-free margarine
50g soft brown sugar

Method

1) Pre-heat the oven to 180C/375F/Gas Mark 5 unless you are using the microwave.

2) Place the apples in a 1 litre oven-proof dish. Sprinkle the apples with the mixed spice and 50g of caster sugar.

3) Place the flour, oats and sugar in a bowl. Rub in the butter **or** margarine. The mixture comes together almost like a cake mixture and will produce a moist crumble. If you prefer a drier crumble add 50g more flour.

4) Spoon the mixture on top of the prepared fruit.

5) Bake in a conventional oven for 15-20 minutes or just 10 minutes on full power in a microwave.

6) Serve on its own or with your choice of custard, cream or ice-cream.

Tip
Try one of these fruit fillings to ring the changes:
Pear and raspberry
rhubarb with the grated rind and juice of an unwaxed orange.
blackcurrants
blackberry and apple
plums with 1 teaspoon cinnamon
gooseberries.

* (If your child has to avoid wheat or barley etc. then make sure the oats you buy are completely pure and not contaminated with other cerals.)

Apple Charlotte

Traditionally made with apple this recipe is easily varied by using 500g of other stewed fruits such as pears, plums, blackberries, cherries, rhubarb or summer fruits.

Serves 6

Ingredients

250g Bramley cooking apples, peeled, cored and cubed
250g eating apples, peeled, cored and cubed
1 unwaxed lemon, rind and juice
½ teaspoon ground cinnamon
Either 75g butter or margarine
      or 75g dairy-free **&/or** soya-free margarine
Either 6 slices of wheat bread
      or 6 slices of gluten-free bread
25-50g caster sugar (to taste)

Method

1) Pre-heat the oven to 180C/375F/Gas 5 and thoroughly grease a 600ml pudding basin.

2) Place the apples in a bowl with the lemon rind and juice, sugar and cinnamon and cook in the microwave for approximately 6 minutes until cooked and softened.

3) Melt the butter **or** margarine in the microwave for approximately 30 seconds.

4) Line the pudding basin with bread, dipping each piece in the melted butter (or margarine) before placing it in the basin. You will need to ensure the slices at the bottom and all around the basin overlap slightly and that you save one dipped slice to act as the lid.

5) Stir the stewed fruit then pour it into the bread-lined basin. Place the last slice of dipped bread on top. At this stage place a small plate on top of the pudding and put a 900g weight on top (if you don't have a cooking weight use a tin, stone or even a book). Leave the weighted pudding in the fridge for 30 minutes to make sure the pudding is compressed and the juices soak into the bread.

6) Bake the pudding in the oven for 30-40 minutes. (If you are using a cooking weight then leave it on top of the pudding for the first 20 minutes before removing it so that the top gets browned.)

7) Turn the pudding out onto a serving plate. Serve hot.

Banoffee Pie

A gooey, golden caramel and banana-filled pastry - it disappears in seconds! The recipe below has a pastry case but use the biscuit crumb base on p180 if preferred.

Serves 6

Ingredients

Base
Either 100g shortcrust pastry
> **or** 100g gluten-free **&/or** dairy-free pastry
> (see p210)

25g cornflour
Either 300ml milk
> **or** 300ml oat, rice or soya milk

Either 25g butter
> **or** 25g dairy-free **&/or** soya-free margarine

50g muscovado sugar
1 teaspoon golden syrup

Topping
2 bananas, peeled
1 lemon, juice

Method

1) Pre-heat the oven to 190C/400F/Gas Mark 6.

2) Roll out the pastry into a circle and line an 18cm flan dish or ring. (The gluten free pastry will be difficult to handle. Either, you will need to use a fish slice to lift it off the work surface, before you press it into the flan dish, or try rolling it out on a board covered with cling film. Then lift the cling film and slide the pastry into the dish.)

3) Place a circle of greaseproof paper in the pastry case and weigh down with baking beans. Place on a high shelf in the oven and bake blind for 10 minutes. Then remove the paper and beans and return to the oven for a further 5 minutes. Once the pastry is firm and golden remove it from the oven and set aside to cool.

4) In a jug mix the cornflour with 2 teaspoon of your choice of milk. Warm the rest of the milk.

5) Melt your choice of butter or margarine, muscovado sugar and golden syrup in a saucepan. Keep stirring all the time until all the ingredients are melted, then mix in the warmed milk. Pour this mixture onto the cornflour paste, stir well and then return it to the pan.

6) Bring the sauce to the boil and simmer until it is thick. Allow it to cool slightly then pour it into the pastry case. Put it in the fridge until it is chilled.

7) Slice the bananas into circles and coat them in lemon juice (to stop the bananas going brown). Place the banana slices on top of the toffee filling and your pie is ready to serve.

Baked Egg Custard

Another simple pudding that bakes in the oven while you get on with the main course, housework or answering e-mails. It is an ideal one to make in advance, refrigerate and serve the next day.

Serves 4

Ingredients

4 eggs
100g caster sugar
½ teaspoon vanilla extract
Either 300ml milk
        or 300ml oat or rice or soya milk
Either 250ml double cream
        or 250ml oat cream or soya cream
½ teaspoon grated nutmeg

Method

1) Pre-heat the oven to 150C/325F/Gas Mark 3.

2) Whisk the eggs, vanilla extract and caster sugar thoroughly (an electric whisk is best). Slowly add the milk while still whisking.

3) Pour into 6 x 150ml ramekin dishes or a 900ml oven-proof dish and sprinkle with grated nutmeg.

4) Stand the dishes in a baking tin which you have already half-filled with water. Bake individual puddings for about 45 minutes. The large pudding will take an hour. The egg custard is cooked when it is set.

5) Chill thoroughly before serving.

Bread and Butter Pudding

A useful way to use up old bread. You can make a richer pudding by replacing 250ml of milk with double cream, oat cream or soya cream. We think oat milk gives the best tasting dairy-free result. If you want to vary the flavour more radically try spreading the buttered bread with jam or marmalade and leave out the sultanas. Serve it hot or cold, with or without cream or custard.

Serves 6

Ingredients

Either 4-6 slices of wheat-bread
         or 4-6 slices gluten-free bread
Either 25g butter or dairy margarine
         or 25g dairy-free **&/or** soya-free margarine
50g sultanas
25g caster sugar
2 teaspoon mixed spice.
3 eggs
Either 400ml milk
         or 400ml oat, rice or soya milk
25g caster sugar

Method

1) Grease a 1.25ml –1.5 litre oven-proof dish.

2) Spread the bread with your choice of butter or margarine. Cut the buttered bread into triangles. Place a layer of triangles in the base of the dish, sprinkle with sultanas, caster sugar and mixed spice. Then arrange the next layer of bread triangles on top and sprinkle again with sultanas, caster sugar and mixed spice. Repeat until the final layer of buttered bread triangles.

3) In a large jug, whisk together the eggs, milk and 25g caster sugar. Pour this mixture over the bread triangles. Place in the fridge for ½ hour.

4) Pre-heat the oven to 150C/325F/Gas Mark 3.

5) Bake the pudding for 40-50 minutes until set and golden brown.

6) Serve hot or cold.

Chocolate and Pear Pancakes

Winter or summer, this is a scrumptious pudding. As an alternative, try layering the pancakes instead of rolling them and then you'll be able to see the pear purée and chocolate spread oozing down over the pancakes.

Serves 4-6

Ingredients
Pancakes
Either 125g plain flour
      or 125g gluten free flour
      or 125g buckwheat flour
½ teaspoon vanilla extract
1 egg
Either 250 ml milk
      or 250 ml oat, rice or soya milk
olive oil to cook

Filling
700g puréed pears
1 teaspoon cinnamon (optional)

Chocolate sauce
Either 200g jar chocolate spread
      or 200g 70%+ dairy-free **&/or** soya-free plain chocolate
      + 250ml double cream **or** oat or soya cream.

Method

1) Place the flour and salt in a mixing bowl. Make a well in the centre and break in the egg and add the vanilla extract.

2) Add half the milk, and mix using a hand whisk. Then add the rest of the milk and whisk again until smooth.

3) Heat a pancake pan or flat frying pan, add 1 tablespoon olive oil and coat the pan with the oil. Once the oil is hot pour in enough batter to coat the base of the pan.

4) Cook the pancake over a moderate heat. When the pancake is brown on one side flip it over and brown the other side.

5) Turn the cooked pancake out onto a plate and spread with 1 tablespoon chocolate sauce*, then, on top of that, spread 3 tablespoons of puréed pear (mixed with cinnamon if using). Roll up the pancake and place in a rectangular serving dish.

6) Continue to cook and fill pancakes until all the batter is used up.

7) Before serving, warm up any remaining chocolate spread or sauce and pour over the top of the row of rolled pancakes.

* Method for chocolate sauce

Melt the chocolate in a bowl over simmering water or place the chocolate in a bowl and melt for 30 seconds in the microwave, keep melting for another ten seconds at a time until the chocolate has melted completely. It is important to keep checking the chocolate is not overheating as it can burn very easily. Stir in the cream of your choice.

175

Cranberry Rice Pudding

Such an easy pudding and so comforting!
For a simpler rice pudding leave out the fruit, or to ring the changes try changing the cranberries to sultanas, cherries, blueberries or whatever takes your fancy.
Dairy, oat and soya milks work best, but if you have to use rice milk it will taste fine but the consistency will be less creamy and more gelatinous. Adding the oat cream or soya cream makes a deliciously creamy rice pudding.

Serves 4-6

Ingredients

Either 25g butter or margarine
       or 25g dairy-free **&/or** soya-free margarine
150g pudding rice
25g sugar
Either 1l milk
       or 1l soya or rice milk
Either 250ml double cream
       or 250ml oat cream or soya cream
1 teaspoon vanilla extract
100g dried cranberries
sprinkling of nutmeg

Method

1) Pre-heat the oven to 150C/325F/Gas Mark 3 and grease a 1.8l ovenproof dish.

2) Place rice, sugar, vanilla extract, your choice of butter or margarine and cranberries in the oven dish. Pour over your choice of milk and cream and stir carefully.

3) Bake in the centre of a pre-heated oven for about 2-3 hours. Stir after the first half-hour. The pudding is cooked when the skin is golden and the pudding is creamy and the rice is soft. Serve it hot or cold, sprinkled with nutmeg.

Slow Cooker Method: Rice pudding can be cooked in a slow cooker. Follow the manufacturer's instructions.

Crunchy Lemon Flan

A lovely sharp, gooey citrus tart. The recipe for the cornflake base works well as an alternative to traditional biscuit crumb bases so the recipe for it is given below and the recipe for the topping is on the facing page.

Serves 6

Ingredients

Base
225g cornflakes, crushed
Either 100g butter or margarine
       or 100g dairy-free **&/or** soya-free margarine
25g soft brown sugar
2 level tablespoon golden syrup

Method

1 Place the margarine, brown sugar and golden syrup in a bowl and heat for 1 minute in the microwave, or over a pan of simmering water, until they have melted. Stir thoroughly. Then mix in the crushed cornflakes.

2 Place the cornflake mixture in a 23cm flan dish and press the mixture down using the back of a spoon. Chill in the fridge for about an hour before adding the topping.

Topping
500ml water
60g cornflour
Either a knob of butter or margarine
          or a knob of dairy-free **&/or** soya-free margarine
2 egg yolks, beaten
2 unwaxed lemons, grated, zest and juice
100g caster sugar
lemon slices to decorate

Method

1) Mix the cornflour to a smooth paste with a little water.

2) Heat the rest of the water with the grated lemon rind to boiling point. (This takes about 2 minutes in the microwave, longer if you are using the hob.) When the water is boiling pour the liquid onto the cornflour and cook for a little longer (1 minute in the microwave) until it is quite thick.

3) Add the slightly beaten eggs and stir well. Then add the lemon juice, your choice of butter or margarine, and sugar. Mix well then cook for a little longer (30 seconds – 1 minute in the microwave) to make sure the egg is cooked. Then mix again thoroughly to make sure the topping has no lumps.

4) Pour onto the chilled crispy cornflake base in the flan case. Refrigerate for a couple of hours before decorating with lemon slices.

5) Serve chilled.

Fruits of the Forest No-cheese Cheesecake

This is such a quick pudding to make and once it is served it disappears even faster. To ring the changes, you can choose any complementary flavour of yoghurt and jelly. Although ready-made biscuits work fine, when I use home-made oat biscuits(see p212) for the base, our family's name for this pudding is ' fabby-flapjack pie'.

Serves 8

Ingredients

Either 150g digestive biscuits, crushed (these contain wheat and dairy)

> **or** 150g Lincoln biscuits (these are dairy-free but contain wheat)
> **or** 150g wheat-free and dairy-free oat biscuits, crushed (or see recipe on p212)

Either 75g butter or margarine

> **or** 75g dairy-free **&/or** soya-free margarine

Either 250ml Fruits of the Forest dairy yoghurt

> + 150ml double cream whipped
> + 135g packet strawberry jelly

or 250ml carton of oat cream

> + 135g packet strawberry jelly
> + 150ml summer fruit juice, boiling

or 250ml Fruits of the Forest soya yoghurt

> +150ml dairy-free cream (oat or soya)
> + 135g packet strawberry jelly

250ml boiling water
50g caster sugar
Fresh strawberries and raspberries to decorate

Method

1) Melt the butter/margarine (either in a saucepan over a low heat or in a microwave proof dish in the microwave for approximately 1 minute on full power).

2) Stir in the crushed biscuits. Press the biscuit mixture into the base of a greased 25cm flan dish. Chill well in the fridge.

3) Melt the jelly in the boiling fruit juice or water. Stir well to dissolve. Then leave to cool until the jelly is setting but not actually set. (The consistency should be thick and sloppy.)

4) In either a blender or food processor's bowl or a large mixing bowl, place the yoghurt (if using), cream, caster sugar and semi-set jelly. Blend well.

5) Pour this mixture over the biscuit base. Then return the pudding to the fridge and chill thoroughly until it is set.

6) To serve decorate with fresh strawberries or raspberries.

Vanilla Ice-cream

While you can easily buy dairy-free and soya-free sorbets in supermarkets it is still hard to find suitable ice-creams. The list of flavour options below makes this recipe really versatile – so much so that for a happy summer an ice-cream maker is the only option.

Serves 6

Ingredients

Either 300 ml double cream +300 ml cow's milk
      or 300 ml oat cream + 300 ml oat milk
      or 300 ml soya cream + 300 ml soya milk
1 vanilla pod (or 1 tablespoon vanilla extract)
6 egg yolks
150g caster sugar

Method

1) Place the milk and cream together in a saucepan. Split the vanilla pod open lengthways, scrape out the seeds and add them to the milk and cream together with the scraped out pod (or add the 1 tablespoon of vanilla extract).

2) Whisk the egg yolks and sugar together until they are thick, creamy, pale in colour and the whisk forms a trail when lifted out of the mixture.

3) Pour on the milk mixture and stir well. Allow to cool, stirring occasionally. Then Remove the vanilla pod if used.

4) *If you have an ice-cream maker:* take the pre-frozen bowl out of the freezer, assemble the machine and start it churning. Pour half of the mixture into the bowl and allow it to freeze and churn for approximately 20-30 minutes following the ice-cream machine manufacturer's instructions. Repeat with the second half of the mixture

5) If you do not have an ice-cream maker: pour the ice-cream into a bowl and place it in the freezer. Remove it every 10-15 minutes and beat it well to break up the ice-crystals as they form. Continue this process until it is set. To soften this ice-cream before serving blitz it quickly in a food processor.

6) Serve on its own or with fresh fruit.

Flavour options

There are numerous ways to ring the changes just bear in mind that freezing dulls flavours so make sure the basic mixture tastes intense before you freeze it.
Try any of these or make up your own:
- 100g puréed fruit such as apple, strawberry, plum, raspberries, blackcurrants, mango, (or a combination)
- 50g cocoa powder **&/or** 100g grated 70% +plain dairy-free **&/or** soya-free
- 100g maple syrup
- 3 unwaxed oranges, grated rind and juice
- 1-2 tablespoons peppermint essence
- 50g chopped crystallized ginger (+100g grated dairy-free **&/or** soya-free plain chocolate)
- 1 teaspoon mixed spice

Meringues

Crisp, sweet and very more-ish. These keep well in an airtight container ready to make a quick pudding. Sandwiched together with melted plain chocolate they are a firm favourite at parties, or you can use all the mixture to make one large meringue and, once it is cooled, spread it with cream and heap with fresh fruit.

Serves 12

Ingredients

200g icing sugar
3 egg whites
Fresh fruit (strawberries, raspberries, peaches)
Cream of your choice

Method

1) Pre-heat the oven to 140C/300F/Gas Mark 2.

2) Line a baking sheet with non-stick parchment paper.

3) Half fill a saucepan with water and heat it to boiling point, then reduce it to a simmer.

4) Place a clean, grease-free bowl over the saucepan (the water must not touch the bowl.) Whisk the egg whites and sugar together in the bowl until the mixture forms soft peaks.

5) Remove the bowl from the heat and continue to whisk until the mixture and bowl have cooled down.

6) Spoon or pipe the mixture into circles on the prepared baking tray (makes 12).

7) Cook for 45 minutes to an hour until the meringues are hard and crisp but still white.

8) Let the meringues cool completely then serve with fresh fruit and the cream of your choice.

Lemon Tart

Served in many restaurants, this popular pudding is easy to reproduce dairy-free, soya-free or wheat-free. It is ideal for special occasions and looks stunning when simply decorated with lemon slices.

Serves 8

Ingredients

Either 250g '00' grade flour + pinch of salt
     or 125g gluten-free flour +125g rice flour
75g caster sugar
3 tablespoons cold water
Either 125g butter
     or 125g dairy-free **&/or** soya-free margarine
7 eggs
175g caster sugar
4 unwaxed lemons, zest and juice

Method

1) Pre-heat the oven to 190C/400F/Gas Mark 6.

2) Place the flour (and salt if using) in a mixing bowl. Add the 75g caster sugar and mix well. Cut your choice of fat into small pieces and rub lightly into the flour, using your fingertips, until the mixture resembles fine breadcrumbs.

3) Add a single, beaten egg and the water. Then bind the mixture together using a knife to form a soft dough that leaves the sides of the bowl clean. Place the dough on a lightly floured work surface and knead lightly into a smooth round ball. Cool for 15 minutes in the refrigerator.

186

4) Roll out the pastry and use to line a 25cm flan tin or dish which has been lightly greased. The gluten-free pastry needs to be approximately 75mm thick. (The gluten free pastry will be difficult to handle. Either, you will need to use a fish slice to lift it off the work surface, before you press it into the flan dish, or try rolling it out on a board covered with cling film. Then lift the cling film and slide the pastry into the dish.)

5) Prick the base of the flan with a fork and bake blind (cover with greaseproof paper weighed down with baking beans) for 10 minutes. Then bake for a further 5 minutes uncovered, until the pastry is dry but not brown. Once cooked remove the flan case and reduce the oven temperature to 150C/325F/Gas Mark 3.

6) Whisk together the remaining 6 eggs and 175 g caster sugar until thick and creamy. (An electric whisk is best.) Stir in the zest and juice of 3 lemons. Then pour into the pastry case.

7) Bake for 35-40 minutes until the filling is springy to touch. Leave to cool, and then chill thoroughly before serving.

Orange Sago Pudding

Forget gran's school sago horror stories. This yummy pudding will be gobbled down in seconds.

While the recipe below works wonderfully, if you are lucky enough to have a slow cooker it's worth the hassle of remembering to put in all the ingredients and switching it on before you go on the afternoon school run. Your reward will be coming home to the fragrant smell of this pudding.

Serves 4

Ingredients

50g sago
Either 850ml full fat milk +150ml double cream
or 850 ml oat, rice or soya milk
+ 150ml oat cream or soya cream
50g caster sugar
2 unwaxed oranges, rind and juice

Method

1) Pre-heat the oven to 180C/375F/Gas Mark 5.

2) Heat the sago, orange juice and rind and your choice of milk and cream in a large saucepan. Bring the liquid to the boil, stirring continuously. Then simmer for about 5 minutes before removing from the heat. Stir in the sugar.

3) Pour the mixture into four small greased, oven-proof ramekin dishes. Stand these dishes in a baking tray half-full of boiling water and place in your pre-heated oven. Bake for 20 minutes until each pudding is light brown.

4) Decorate each pudding with a thin slice of orange. Serve hot or cold.

Slow cooker method: Switch the slow cooker onto its high setting. Then place all the ingredients in the pot and stir well. The pudding will need to cook for approximately two hours on full power setting until it is thick and creamy.

Queen of Puddings

Lovely hot or cold - it never fails to please, and is a great way to use up bread that is too dry for sandwiches but still fresh enough to turn into breadcrumbs.

Serves 4-6

Ingredients

Either 400ml milk
>   or 400ml oat, rice or soya milk

Either 25g butter
>   **or** 25g dairy-free **&/or** soya-free margarine

1 unwaxed lemon, grated rind
2 eggs, separated
50g caster sugar
Either 75g breadcrumbs
>   **or** 75g gluten-free breadcrumbs

2 tablespoons good quality strawberry or raspberry jam

Method

1) Pre-heat your oven to 180C/375F/Gas Mark 5.

2) Warm your choice of milk, together with the butter/margarine and lemon rind.

3) Lightly whisk the egg yolks with half the sugar. Then pour on the warmed milk mixture and stir well.

4) Pour the egg custard over the breadcrumbs and mix well. Transfer this into a greased 1 litre oven proof dish and leave to stand for 15 minutes. Then bake for 20-30 minutes until set.

5) Spread the cooked pudding with jam.

6) In a clean, dry, grease-free bowl whisk the egg whites until stiff, add 25g of caster sugar, whisk again, then add the final 25g of caster sugar.

7) Pile the whisked egg whites on top of the jam and bake for a further 5-10 minutes until the meringue is slightly browned on top.

8) Serve hot or cold.

Sultana and Carrot Pudding

The carrots sweeten, brighten and moisten this fragrant, spongy pudding – and you have sneaked another portion of vegetables on to your children's plates. Perfect with custard. Perfect without.

Serves 4

Ingredients

Either 50g breadcrumbs
       or 50g gluten-free breadcrumbs
50g fine oatmeal
25g porridge oats*
50g caster sugar
100g carrots, peeled and grated
½ teaspoon grated nutmeg
½ teaspoon cinnamon
3 tablespoons orange juice
1 unwaxed orange, juiced and grated rind
100g sultanas
2 eggs, separated

* (If your child has to avoid wheat or barley etc. then make sure the oats you buy are completely pure and not contaminated with other cerals.)

Method

1) Mix together the breadcrumbs, oatmeal, oats, caster sugar, grated carrot and spices.

2) Stir in the sultanas, orange rind and juice and beat in the egg yolks.

3) In a clean, grease-free bowl whisk the egg whites until stiff. Then, using a figure of eight action, fold them into the orange mixture.

4) Pour into a greased 900ml microwavable pudding basin. Cook on **full** power for 4-5 minutes. It is cooked when a skewer is inserted and comes out clean.

5) Run a knife around the bowl and turn the pudding out onto a serving plate. Serve hot.

12: Tea Time and Treats

Banana Cake

If your supermarket has a glut of bananas this is a brilliant way to make the most of them. Even if there's no glut this cake is so light and yummy you'll want to make it frequently. You can vary the taste by using 1 teaspoon of mixed spice instead of the vanilla extract.

Serves 8-10

Ingredients

3 large eggs
150g caster sugar
Either 100g butter or margarine
        or 100g dairy-free **&/or** soya-free margarine
Either 150ml milk
        or 150 ml oat, rice or soya milk
2 ripe bananas, peeled
2 teaspoon vanilla extract
3 teaspoon baking powder
100g polenta
100g rice flour

Method

1) Pre-heat the oven to 180C/375F/Gas Mark 5. Either take a 20cm cake tin and grease and then dust it with rice flour or line it with grease proof paper.

2) Whisk the eggs with the sugar until the mixture is thick and creamy and the whisk leaves a trail when it is lifted out.

3) Put the butter/margarine and milk in a microwave proof jug and heat in the microwave for one minute.

4) Add the bananas and vanilla extract to the whisked eggs and mix well.

5) Add the baking powder to the milk mixture then pour this onto the banana and egg mixture. Add the polenta and rice flour and mix well.

6) Pour into the prepared cake tin. Bake in a pre-heated oven for 20-30 minutes until golden brown, springy to touch and a skewer inserted into the cake comes out clean.

7) Cool on a wire rack before serving.

Biscuits Galore!

We bake biscuits regularly – the children love helping and since we all enjoy munching the wheat-free, dairy and soya-free version, everyone gets to benefit from eating a healthier biscuit than the additive-loaded, refined supermarket versions.

Vary the basic recipe by deciding which flavour you want to add from the list below. We find that the results are better if we use more flavouring with gluten-free flour than we would normally use with wheat flour.

Makes 16

Ingredients
Basic biscuit mix
Either 125g butter *or* margarine
      or 125g dairy-free **&/or** soya-free margarine
100g caster sugar
2 egg yolks
Either 225g plain flour, sifted
      or 300g gluten-free flour, sifted

Flavour options:
Add <u>one</u> of these to the basic mix:

- 2-3 teaspoon grated unwaxed lemon rind (use an unwaxed lemon)
- 2-3 teaspoon grated unwaxed orange rind
- ½ - 1 teaspoon vanilla extract
- 1 teaspoon cinnamon
- 1 teaspoon mixed spice
- For chocolate flavoured biscuits: replace 25g of plain flour or 50g of the gluten-free flour with the same amount of dairy **&/or** soya-free drinking chocolate powder

Method

1) Cream the butter or margarine with the sugar and flavouring option (but not the drinking chocolate powder) until light and smooth.

2) Gradually beat in the egg yolks, and then mix in the flour (and drinking chocolate powder if you are using it.)

3) Knead the dough lightly then form into a ball. If it is very dry and crumbly add 1-2 tablespoons of your usual milk. Then bring the mixture together to form a ball and place on a lightly floured plate. Cover it with cling film and chill in the fridge for 30 minutes until firm.

4) Pre-heat the oven to 170C/350F/Gas Mark 4.

5) Using a floured rolling pin roll out the dough on a floured surface to approximately 1cm thick.

6) Take a 6cm round cutter, and cut out the biscuits. (If the dough becomes sticky while you are handling it then return it to the fridge for a few minutes).

7) Place on a greased baking sheet and bake in a pre-heated oven for about 10 minutes. (When cooked, the gluten-free biscuits will look very pale compared to the wheat version.) Then cool on a wire tray.

8) Once cooled, these biscuits can be decorated with icing for special occasions.

Bread Pudding

Bread pudding – sold by my grandparent's local baker, made by my mother on a Thursday… it brings back lots of memories. The happiest are of munching lightly spiced fruity mouthfuls still warm from the oven, though, of course, some people prefer theirs eaten as a pudding with custard. If you want to make the bread pudding dairy-free then choosing oat milk really improves the flavour.

Serves 6

Ingredients

Either 225g wheat bread
       or 225g gluten-free bread
Either 300ml milk
       or 300ml oat, rice or soya milk
Either 50g butter
       or dairy-free **&/or** soya- free margarine
75g soft brown sugar
2 teaspoon mixed spice
1 egg, beaten
150g sultanas
½ teaspoon nutmeg

Method

1) Grease a 1.25 –1.5 litre ovenproof dish.

2) Break up the bread into small pieces and place them in a mixing bowl. Pour over the milk and leave to stand for ½ hr so it all soaks in. Then stir well till the mixture is smooth.

3) Pre-heat the oven to 150C/325F/Gas Mark 3.

4) Melt the butter or margarine in the microwave for 30 second or in a small saucepan. Pour on to the bread mixture and stir well.

5) Add the sugar, mixed spice, sultanas and beaten egg. Mix well to ensure that there are no lumps.

6) Pour the mixture into the greased, ovenproof dish and sprinkle with nutmeg. Bake in a pre-heated oven for 1 to 1½ hours until set and firm.

7) Serve hot as a pudding with custard, cream or ice-cream, or cold as a cake.

Chocolate Biscuit Cake

Sweet and more-ish, this is lovely as a pudding or tea-time treat. You can vary the flavour by adding glacé cherries or replacing the vanilla extract with grated orange rind, or mixed spice or cinnamon. Alternatively you can ring the changes by using different-flavoured biscuits such as ginger.

Serves 8

Ingredients

225g 70%+ plain dairy-free **&/or** soya-free chocolate, broken into pieces
Either 100g butter or margarine
    or 100g dairy-free **&/or** soya-free margarine
Either 397g can sweetened condensed milk
    or 250ml oat cream or soya cream
Either 250g lincoln biscuits
    or 250g gluten-free biscuits (see p196)
50g sultanas
1 teaspoon vanilla extract

Method

1) Place the chocolate pieces, butter or margarine into a glass bowl with the condensed milk or soya cream or oat cream.

2) Heat the mixture in the microwave for approximately one minute (or over a pan of simmering water) till the chocolate and butter or margarine has melted then stir slowly to mix everything together. Cook for another minute and stir again so that all the ingredients are thoroughly combined.

3) Break up the biscuits into small pieces. Then add to the chocolate mixture together with the sultanas and vanilla extract. Mix well.

4) Press the mixture into a 20cm square dish. Refrigerate and chill until firm then cut into slices and serve.

Chocolate Chip Cakes

This is a really useful small-cake recipe. You can vary it by replacing the chocolate chips with the same quantity of sultanas, currants, chopped dates, chopped glacé cherries or even crystallized ginger. For a really light cake, use margarine and mix in a food mixer. Children especially love eating these still warm from the oven.

Makes 12

Ingredients

Either 100g butter or margarine
    or 100g dairy-free **&/or** soya-free margarine
100g caster sugar
2 eggs, beaten
1 teaspoon vanilla extract
Either 50g milk, chocolate chips
    or 50g plain, chocolate chips
    or 50g 70% + plain dairy-free,
    &/or soya-free chocolate, chopped
Either 100g self raising flour
    or 100g gluten-free flour +1 teaspoon gluten-free
    baking powder + ½ teaspoon xanthan gum
12 paper cases

Method

1) Pre-heat the oven to 180C/375F/Gas Mark 5 and place 12 paper cases into patty tins.

2) Cream the fat and sugar together until pale and fluffy.

3) Then add the egg little by little, together with the vanilla extract. Beat well after each addition.

4) In a separate bowl, mix your choice of chocolate chips or chopped chocolate with the flour (and baking powder and xanthan gum if used). Fold into the cake mixture.

5) Using a tablespoon two-thirds fill the paper cases with the cake mixture.

6) Bake in the pre-heated oven for approximately 10 minutes. Although the gluten-free cakes will be very pale in colour, the cooked cakes will be springy to touch.

7) Serve straight out of the oven, cooled slightly.

Flapjacks

A treat for all the family to enjoy. If you bake these in the microwave then they remain soft and slightly gooey - a nice change to the firmer oven-baked flapjacks. Adding 1-2 tablespoons of drinking chocolate powder gives the flapjack a lovely chocolate flavour when you fancy a change.

Makes 12 pieces

Ingredients

Either 100g butter or margarine
        or 100g dairy-free **&/or** soya-free margarine
100g soft brown sugar
6 tablespoon golden syrup
250g porridge oats*

* *(If your child has to avoid wheat or barley etc. then make sure the oats you buy are completely pure and not contaminated with other cereals.)*

Method

1) Grease a rectangular oven-proof dish that measures approximately 18cm x 23cm.

2) Place the butter or margarine, syrup and sugar in a pan and heat gently till the ingredients have melted. Alternatively place the ingredients in a glass bowl and cook in a microwave oven (it takes about one minute). Stir well. Then add the oats and mix well.

3) Pour into the prepared dish and press down well.

4) Either bake in the microwave for 3½ minutes or in a pre-heated oven at 170C/350F/Gas Mark 4 for 20-25 minutes.

5) Leave to cool then cut into rectangles. Serve.

6) Any remaining flapjack must be stored in an air-tight container.

Gingerbread Men (or Women!)

My earliest memory of baking is standing on a stool next to my dough-covered dad. I am happily pushing sultana eyes and glacé cherry mouths into ginger-bread men. And now I get to do it all over again with my own kids! (Except this generation seem to prefer using tubes of garish-coloured icing, little sweets and silver balls to decorate them.)
By changing the cutter shape and decorations this recipe is a good standby for rainy afternoons. Your children will love creating Christmas trees, snowmen, Halloween spider's webs, fancy fireworks – the only limit is their imaginations (and your time and patience!)
Finished biscuits need to be kept in an airtight tin.

Makes approximately 24

Ingredients

Either 250g plain flour
      or 250g gluten-free flour
1 teaspoon gluten-free baking powder
Either 100g butter
      or 100g dairy-free **&/or** soya-free margarine
1teaspoon ginger
2 tablespoon golden syrup
100g soft brown sugar.
edible decorations: tubes of coloured icing, gluten- free **&/or** dairy-free sweets, icing flowers, silver balls etc.
or currants and glacé cherries

Method

1) Pre-heat the oven to 180C/375 F/Gas Mark 5.

2) Line two baking sheets with baking parchment. (This makes lifting off the cooked biscuits, without breaking them, so much easier.)

3) Rub the fat into the flour until the mixture resembles fine breadcrumbs.

4) Stir in the ginger and brown sugar thoroughly. Then, spoon in the golden syrup and continue mixing until a soft dough ball forms.

5) Place the dough on a small plate and cover with cling film. Chill in the fridge for 30 minutes.

6) After flouring the work surface and rolling pin, roll the dough out to 1cm thick. Using a small gingerbread man cutter, cut out approximately 24 gingerbread men. Space them out on the baking sheets.

7) Cook the biscuits in a pre-heated oven for 10 minutes until they are firm but do not allow them to brown. Remove the tray from the oven and leave for 10 minutes before transferring them onto a cooling rack.

8) Decorate the gingerbread men with tubes of coloured icing etc. (E.g. Make 2 icing dots for the eyes and add a smiling mouth and belt) or use currants and glacé cherries.

Chocolate Brownies

Who doesn't love chocolate fudge brownies? The rice flour version works just as well as the wheat version – if not better - so the whole family can enjoy the same recipe.

Makes 12 pieces

Ingredients

Either 150g butter
      or 150g dairy-free **&/or** soya-free margarine
200g 70%+dairy-free **&/or** soya-free plain chocolate,
      broken into pieces
350g soft brown sugar
4 eggs, beaten
1 teaspoon vanilla extract
Either 150g plain flour
      or 150g rice flour
2 teaspoon baking powder

Method

1) Pre-heat the oven to 180C/375F/Gas Mark 5 and grease or line a 28cm square, shallow baking tin.

2) Place your choice of butter or margarine in a glass bowl and add the broken chocolate pieces. *Either* place the bowl over a pan of boiling water and stir until the chocolate and fat have melted, *or* place the bowl in a microwave and heat for 1-2 minutes till melted. Do not stir the chocolate too much when melting it as this causes it to thicken which means you will not achieve the smooth glossy result you are aiming for.

3) In another bowl, mix together the eggs, sugar and vanilla essence. Pour this into the chocolate mixture, then add the flour and baking powder and mix thoroughly.

4) Pour the mixture into the prepared tin. Bake in the pre-heated oven for approximately 30 minutes. The brownies are cooked when a skewer, placed in the centre of the tin comes out clean. Cool and cut into slices to serve.

5) Freeze the slices that are not eaten for another day and de-frost as needed. This makes the chocolate fudge brownie taste really fresh and easy to pop into lunch boxes.

Jam Tarts

Jam tarts are traditionally English and children still love making them today - rolling out pastry and cutting out the circles is easy for even the smallest members of the family. The quality of the jam makes all the difference to how good they taste – we've suggested strawberry but vary the flavour to suit yourself.

Makes 12-14

Ingredients

Either 200g plain flour + pinch of salt
    or 100g gluten-free plain flour +100g rice flour
Either 100g butter
    or 100g dairy-free **&/or** soya-free margarine
1 egg, beaten
2-3 tablespoons cold water
1 jar of good quality strawberry jam

Method

1) 1 Pre-heat the oven to 190C/400F/Gas Mark 6. Grease 14 patty tins.

2) Place your choice of flour (and salt if used) in a mixing bowl. Then cut the fat into small pieces and rub lightly into the flour, using your fingertips, until the mixture resembles fine breadcrumbs.

3) Add the beaten egg and water. Then bind the mixture, using a knife, so that it clings together leaving the sides of the bowl clean. Knead lightly into a smooth round ball.

4) Roll out the pastry, cut into 8cm circles and use to line 12-14 patty tins. (N.B. The gluten-free pastry will need to be kept quite thick. The gluten free pastry will be difficult to handle. Either, you will need to use a fish slice to lift it off the work surface, before you press it into the flan dish, or try rolling it out on a board covered with cling film. Then lift the cling film and slide the pastry into the patty tins.)

5) Place a tablespoon of jam into each pastry case.

6) Bake for 15-20 minutes. (The gluten-free pastry will remain very pale.)

7) Cool on a wire rack before serving.

Oat Biscuits

Tasty and transportable – these everyday biscuits are a hit with children of every age. For special occasions they are extra nice topped with melted dark chocolate rather than sprinkled with caster sugar.

Makes 16

Ingredients

225g rolled porridge oats* (plus extra for rolling out)
Either 100g self raising flour
+ pinch of salt
+ 1 tablespoon baking powder
       or 100g gluten-free flour
       +1 teaspoon gluten-free baking powder
Either 50g butter
       or 50g dairy-free **&/or** soya-free margarine
125g caster sugar

(If your child has to avoid wheat or barley etc. then make sure the oats you buy are completely pure and not contaminated with other cerals.)

Method

1) Pre-heat the oven to 150C/325F/Gas Mark 3 and grease a baking sheet.

2) Mix together the oats, your choice of flour (and salt if used) and baking powder.

3) Rub in your choice of butter or margarine. Then stir in 100g caster sugar. Add 2 tablespoon water and bind to make a firm dough (add a little more water if needed).

4) Scatter some oats on the work surface, then roll out the dough to 6mm thick. Using a 6cm cutter, press out 16 rounds and place on the baking sheet. Cook for 20-25 minutes until the biscuits are browned at the edges.

5) Leave to cool on the baking sheet, then transfer to a wire rack.

6) Sprinkle with caster sugar for decoration before serving.

Rich Chocolate Cake

This makes a fantastic birthday cake or a really rich cake for afternoon tea. Of course, the higher the cocoa content of the plain chocolate, the richer the cake will be. For an adult-only version, you can replace the vanilla in the cake ingredients with one tablespoon of rum, and add another tablespoon of rum to the chocolate icing.

Serves 8

Ingredients for the cake
225g 70%+ plain dairy-free **&/or** soya-free chocolate
    broken into pieces
2 tablespoons strong black coffee
1 teaspoon vanilla essence
Either 100g unsalted butter cut into pieces
    or 100g dairy-free **&/or** soya-free spread
4 eggs, separated
100g caster sugar
Either 75g plain flour
or 75g gluten-free plain flour

Ingredients for the chocolate icing
Either 150ml double cream
    or 150ml oat or soya cream
150g 70%+plain dairy-free **&/or** soya-free chocolate
    broken into pieces
25g icing sugar
1 teaspoon vanilla extract

To decorate:
70%+plain dairy-free **&/or** soya-free chocolate, grated
sieved icing sugar.

Method

1) Pre-heat oven to 180C/375F/Gas Mark 5 and thoroughly grease and flour a ring mould.

2) Place the chocolate, coffee and vanilla essence in a large glass bowl and melt the chocolate (either in the microwave for one minute, or over a pan of hot water). Once the chocolate has melted, stir the mixture gently until it is smooth and thoroughly blended.

3) Add your choice of butter or margarine pieces to the mixture and mix well. Then stir in the egg yolks, sugar and the flour.

4) In a clean, grease-free bowl, whisk the egg whites until stiff, then gently fold a third of them into the chocolate cake mixture. Add the remaining egg whites taking care not to over mix (or you will lose all the air that helps the cake rise.) Use a metal spoon and a figure of eight action.

5) Pour the mixture into the mould and bake in a pre-heated oven for 45 minutes until the cake is springy to touch. (A cake skewer should come out clean when inserted into the middle of the cake.)

6) Before decorating, leave the cake to cool for 5 minutes in the tin. Then place it onto a wire rack.

To decorate:

Pour your choice of cream into a saucepan and heat until it is almost boiling. Remove from the heat and stir in the broken chocolate, vanilla and icing sugar. Continue stirring until all the chocolate has melted. As the mixture cools it becomes thick and smooth. Once it has cooled spread the chocolate icing over the cake and decorate with grated chocolate and icing sugar.

Scones

English summer treats, winter walk rewards. These scones are best eaten on the day they are cooked (and preferably only two minutes after), spread with butter or dairy-free margarine and jam.

What seems like a lot of raising agent results in really light scones rather than the doughier results of more traditional gluten-free recipes.

Makes 12

Ingredients

Either 500g plain flour
      or 500g gluten-free plain flour
2 teaspoons bicarbonate of soda
½ teaspoon salt
4 ½ teaspoons cream of tartar
Either 75g butter
      or 75g dairy-free **&/or** soya-free margarine
Either 250ml milk
      or 250ml oat, rice or soya milk
2 large eggs
50g caster sugar

Method

1) Pre-heat the oven to 190C/400F/Gas Mark 6. Grease and flour a baking sheet.

2) Sift the flour, bicarbonate of soda, cream of tartar and salt into a mixing bowl. Then rub in the butter or margarine until the mixture resembles fine breadcrumbs.

3) Stir in the caster sugar. Make a well in the middle of the bowl. Pour in the milk and beaten eggs and mix well.

4) Turn out onto a floured surface and briefly knead the dough lightly (don't overdo it or the scones will be heavy).

5) Roll out the dough to 3cm thick. Use a small round cutter or glass and cut out round scones *or* just slice up the dough into triangles or fingers. Place on the greased baking sheet.

6) Cook in a pre-heated oven for 10 minutes until risen and slightly golden. (Don't overcook or the scones will become hard.) Cool on a wire rack.

7) Freeze any leftover scones, then warm them through again before serving.

Spicy Pear Cake

Moist, fruity and fragrant – this cake is wonderful eaten still warm from the oven on cold, wintry days, or fridge-cold accompanied by ice-cream as the perfect ending to a lazy summer lunch.

This recipe works just as well with cooking apple instead of pear.

Serves 8

Ingredients

2 large eggs
200g caster sugar
Either 100g butter or margarine
       or 100g dairy-free **&/or** soya-free margarine
Either 150 ml milk
       or 150ml oat, rice or soya milk
Either 100g plain flour
       or 100g gluten-free flour
75g buckwheat flour
1 teaspoon mixed spice
3 teaspoon gluten-free baking powder
3 large or 4 smaller pears, peeled, cored and sliced
25g caster sugar to sprinkle on the baked cake

For serving
Maple syrup to drizzle on each slice before serving

Method

1) Pre-heat the oven to 180C/375F/Gas Mark 5.

2) Line a 25cm diameter round cake tin with grease-proof paper.

3) Whisk the eggs and 200g of caster sugar in a bowl until the mixture is thick and creamy. The whisk should leave a trail behind when it is lifted out of the mixture.

4) **Either** put the butter or margarine and your choice of milk into a pan gently stirring as the fat melts bringing the mixture to the boil.

5) **Or** put the butter or margarine and your choice of milk into a microwave-proof bowl and heat on full power for approximately 1 ½ minutes until the liquid starts boiling. Remove and stir.

6) Add the still boiling liquid to the whisked eggs and sugar. Stir in a figure of eight with a metal spoon.

7) Sieve the flour, baking powder and mixed spice together. Then fold it carefully into the liquid, ensuring there are no lumps.

8) Pour the batter into the prepared tin. Arrange the sliced pears in a neat pattern on top.

9) Bake in a pre-heated oven for 20-25 minutes until well risen, springy and golden in colour. Insert a cake tester to check it is done – it should come out clean.

10) Before cutting, sprinkle the cake top with caster sugar. Then drizzle maple syrup over each slice as you serve it.

Sunshine Cake

For gloomy winter days this golden, yellow cake scented with oranges and kept moist by the surprise ingredient (courgette) is unbeatable. Not only does the hidden vegetable add vitamins, moisture *and* improve the cake's texture, it also has an undetectable taste and lowers the cake's glycaemic index.
Oh, and it tastes fab!

Serves 12-16

Ingredients

Either 200g butter
            or 200g dairy-free **&/or** soya-free margarine
200g caster sugar
1 large courgette, washed and grated
1 large unwaxed orange, grated zest and juice
3 eggs, beaten
1 ½ teaspoon baking powder
1 ½ teaspoon bicarbonate of soda
200g polenta

Method

1) Pre-heat oven to 180C/375F/Gas Mark 5.

2) Grease and line with greaseproof paper, a 25cm square cake tin.

3) Cream the butter or margarine and caster sugar together. Then add the eggs, grated courgette, orange juice and zest. Mix thoroughly.

4) Stir in the polenta, baking powder and bicarbonate of soda and mix well. Pour the cake mixture into the prepared cake tin.

5) Bake in a pre-heated oven for 25 minutes till golden brown, springy to touch and a cake tester comes out clean.

6) Cool on a wire rack. Serve in slices. Refrigerate any remaining slices.

Spice Cake

The high protein gram flour in this cake makes it especially useful if your child is on a milk-free and soya-free diet. Sometimes it is hard to persuade a child to eat more meat but a piece of cake is always welcome.

Serves 8-10

Ingredients

100g *gram flour
1 egg, beaten
Either 100g butter
          or dairy-free **&/or** soya-free margarine
100g Demerara sugar
2 teaspoons baking powder
2 teaspoons vanilla extract
1 teaspoon cinnamon
1 teaspoon nutmeg

Anyone with an allergy to nuts should avoid gram flour because it is made from chick peas.

Method

1) Pre-heat oven to 170C/350F/Gas Mark 4 and grease and flour (with gram flour) a 20cm square cake tin.

2) Cream the butter or margarine and Demerara sugar together then add the vanilla extract and beaten egg.

3) In a separate bowl mix the gram flour and spices, before adding it spoon by spoon to the other ingredients. Mix well.

4) Pour the cake mixture into the prepared cake tin and bake in a pre-heated oven for 20 – 30 minutes until the cake is lightly browned and a cake tester comes out clean.

5) Cool and serve in slices.

13: Kids in the Kitchen

Welcome to your very own section of the book. All the recipes in this section are a) yummy b) good for chefs who are just starting out.

When you want to cook make sure an adult is standing by ready to help you deal with hot or sharp things (blood doesn't improve the flavour of any of these recipes!). Then as long as you follow the rules below you will be a safe cook and the rest of your family will enjoy you being in the kitchen too!

Top Chef's Rules:

1) Check that it is okay to cook today.

2) Before you begin, read the recipe carefully all the way through. Make sure you understand what you have to do.

3) Check that you have <u>all</u> the ingredients and equipment you need *before* you start.

4) **Always wash your hands with soap and warm water before you start cooking and after handling meat or fish**. That gets rid of the germs. Wear an apron and tie back your hair (if it is long) to keep you clean and the food fluff and hair-free.

5) Before you start cooking clean the work surface using a clean cloth and a kitchen cleaning spray.

6) Wash fruit, vegetables and salad ingredients carefully in cold water before you use them.

7) Keep all refrigerated foods in the refrigerator until you need them. Make sure you return them to the refrigerator when you have finished using them.

8) Wash meat and fish under cold, running water before you use them.

9) Use a separate chopping board and knife to prepare raw meat and fish. (You don't want any germs from them getting on the fruit and vegetables). Use a different chopping board and knife to prepare ready-cooked food or fruit and vegetables.

10) **Take care when you use a knife.** Always ask an adult to help you. Remember to hold the knife so that the sharp blade points downwards. Then cut downwards on to a chopping board. Make sure you always keep your fingers away from the sharp blade.

11) **Always ask an adult to help you use the cooker** and wear oven gloves when moving hot food.

12) Measure and weigh out your ingredients accurately or the recipe will not work.

13) Clean up carefully at the end of your cooking session. Wash and dry the equipment before putting it away. (If you don't clean up properly you may not be allowed back in the kitchen! Adults hate cleaning up messy kitchens)

14) Don't leave cooked or half-eaten food out in the kitchen. Once it has cooled, put cooked food away in air-tight containers or cover it with cling film and put it in the refrigerator.

15) Enjoy yourself while cooking in the kitchen but be safe and sensible at all times.

I've read the rules and I am going to follow them every time I cook:

Signed_____

Chicken and Vegetable Kebabs

This is a recipe that you can vary as much as you like by changing the meat to frying steak, lamb steak or pork fillet, and changing the vegetables to chunks of pepper, onion or even aubergine. They make a great meal served with salad or popped into pitta breads with leaves and sauces.

Serves 4-6

Ingredients

2 skinless chicken breasts, washed
1 small packet cherry tomatoes, washed
1 small packet baby sweetcorn, washed
1 small packet button mushrooms, wiped clean
2 courgettes, washed
4 tablespoons olive oil

Method

1) If you are using wooden skewers, soak them for 30 minutes in cold water. (This stops them from burning and catching fire while the kebabs cook!). Metal skewers are safer but you must remember to use oven gloves to handle them when the kebabs are cooking as the skewers get very hot.

2) Cut the chicken into 2 ½ cm cubes. Place on a clean plate. Clean your knives, chopping board and work surface with an anti bacterial spray and wash your hands with a disinfectant soap before moving on to the next step.

3) Cut the baby sweetcorn in half and the courgettes into 2 ½ cm slices.

4) Thread each skewer using up all your ingredients: you could start with mushroom then sweetcorn, then chicken, then tomato, then courgette or any pattern you like.

5) Use a pastry brush to brush each kebab with the olive oil. Then place them on a grill rack and grill or barbecue over a high heat. (Ask your adult helper to help you with this.)

6) Serve hot or cold.

Fruity Savoury Salad

The ingredients below work well together but feel free to swap in your favourite fruit and vegetables!

Serves 4

Ingredients

1 Gem lettuce
¼ cucumber
1 dessert apple (Royal Gala or Pink Lady)
1 ripe peach
10 seedless black grapes
6 cherry tomatoes
½ packet cress

Method

1) Peel off the lettuce leaves. Rip them up into small pieces, wash well in cold water and then dry off before placing in a large serving bowl.

2) Wash the cucumber, apple, grapes and tomatoes.

3) Slice the cucumber as thinly as possible then place in the serving bowl on top of the lettuce.

4) Remove the core from the apple, slice the apple into small pieces and add to the salad.

5) Peel the peach, cut it into small pieces and add to the salad.

6) Sprinkle the salad with tomatoes and grapes.

7) Cut the cress with a pair of scissors and sprinkle over the salad. Now it is ready to serve.

Pitta Bread Sandwiches

Sandwiches – great for lunchboxes, tea, party spreads or to satisfy those midnight munchies. Have fun creating your own pitta fillings but the ideas below should keep your family happy for quite some time!

Serves 4-6

Ingredients

Either 1 packet pitta bread
      or 1 packet gluten-free pitta bread
+ your choice of the following fillings:

Method

1) Warm the pitta bread in the toaster.

2) Ask for an adult's help when removing them from the toaster and splitting them open as they contain very hot steam.

3) Fill with one of the fillings on the following pages.

BLT

Thinly sliced iceberg lettuce
Thinly sliced tomatoes
2 slices smoked bacon, cooked, chopped
3 basil leaves, chopped
1 tablespoon mayonnaise

Method

1) Spread the inside of the pitta bread with mayonnaise.

2) Fill with sliced, lettuce, tomato, basil and bacon. Then serve.

Grilled Chicken and Salsa

1 grilled chicken breast, chopped
Thinly sliced lettuce
1 tablespoon salsa
1 tablespoon mayonnaise

Method

1) Spread the inside of the pitta bread with mayonnaise.

2) Add the sliced lettuce and chopped chicken. Then drizzle over with salsa and serve.

Salmon and Cucumber

1 small tin of salmon, mashed
lettuce, thinly sliced
tomato, thinly sliced
½ lemon, juice
Thin slices of cucumber

Method

1) Spread the inside of the pitta bread with mayonnaise.

2) Add the sliced lettuce, tomato and cucumber. Then top with mashed salmon. Finally squeeze the lemon's juice over the filling and serve.

Tuna and Sweetcorn

1x 170g tin tuna fish
lettuce, thinly sliced
50g sweetcorn
1 teaspoon fresh thyme, chopped
2 tablespoon mayonnaise

Method

1) Sprinkle the pitta with lettuce.

2) Mix together the tuna, sweetcorn, chopped thyme and mayonnaise in a bowl.

3) Fill the pitta with the tuna and sweetcorn filling and serve.

Sardine and Tomato Oatcakes

These make a very tasty TV snack.

Serves 4

Ingredients

150g Scottish oatcakes
1 x 125g tin sardines in oil
2 tablespoons mayonnaise
ground pepper
2 tomatoes, thinly sliced

Method

1) Ask an adult to open the tin of sardines and place them in a clean bowl.

2) Mash the sardines well with a fork. (You can eat everything that is in the tin. Mash up the bones with the fish – not only are they very good for you, they taste great too!)

3) Add the mayonnaise and a twist or two of pepper. Mix well.

4) Spoon onto the oatcakes, top with a slice of tomato. Place on a serving plate. Serve.

Guacamole Dip with Tortilla Chips

Check no one is allergic to avocados before cooking this delicious snack which is also packed full of vitamins. If you would like a really spicy guacamole then try adding a finely chopped fresh chilli – but remember to keep your fingers away from your eyes or they will really sting!

Serves 6

Ingredients

2 large ripe avocados
1 lemon, juice
½ - 1 ½ teaspoon chilli powder
salt and freshly ground pepper
1 packet natural Tortilla chips (Check your brand is dairy-free **&/or** wheat free **&/or** soya-free.)

Method

1) Cut the avocados in half. Remove the stones and throw them away. Then scoop out the avocado flesh and put into a clean bowl. Mash it with a fork until it is a smooth paste.

2) Squeeze the lemon and pour the juice over the avocado. Add the chilli powder (use ½ teaspoon if you like it mild, 1 teaspoon for strong and 1 ½ teaspoon for very strong.) Season with a little salt and pepper. Then mix until smooth. (In the summer you may wish to chill the guacamole in the fridge for a half hour before serving it.)

3) Place the avocado mix in a small bowl on the centre of a plate. Sprinkle the tortilla chips around the bowl and you are ready to dip and munch.

Tuna and Mayo Jacket Potatoes

This recipe works just as well with cooked chicken instead of tuna.

Serves 2 - 4

Ingredients

2 large baking potatoes
185g tin of tuna chunks, drained
2 spring onions, finely chopped (using scissors)
25g tinned sweetcorn
2-3 tablespoon mayonnaise
Either 15g butter or margarine
       or 15g dairy-free **&/or** soya-free margarine

Method

1) Wash and scrub the potatoes. Then prick them well with a fork. Cook in the microwave for approximately 10 minutes until soft.

2) Mix together the drained tuna, finely chopped spring onion and sweetcorn. Add the mayonnaise and stir well.

3) Cut the cooked potatoes in half and place on the serving plate. Use a fork to ruffle up the potato and add the butter or margarine.

4) Pile the tuna and mayonnaise mixture on top.

5) Serve with chopped lettuce and sliced tomatoes and cucumber.

Fruit in Jelly

Remember to make this at least four hours before you want to eat it!

Serves 4

Ingredients

1 x 135g packet strawberry jelly
570ml water
75g frozen fruits of the forest.

Method

1) Break the jelly into cubes and place it into a measuring jug that is safe to go in the microwave. Cover the jelly with water. (This will be up to about 250mls.)

2) Place the jug in the microwave and cook for 1 minute. Then check to see if the jelly has all dissolved. If it has not dissolved, then cook it for another 30 seconds. (Do not cook for more than this in case the jelly boils because then it will never set.)

3) Take the jug out of the microwave and stir the jelly well until all the jelly cubes are completely dissolved. Then add the rest of the water filling the jug up to 570ml.

4) Add the fruit to the jelly and stir well.

5) Pour into your serving dish and cover with cling film. Place in the fridge until it is firm and set. (Remember the coolest part of the fridge is the bottom so the jelly will set fastest if you put it there.)

6) Serve straight from the fridge.

Strawberry Fruit Mousse

This pudding is quick to prepare and easily varied by choosing different flavoured jellies and yoghurts. The only fruits to avoid are fresh pineapple, kiwi and papaya as they will stop the jelly from setting. The oat cream version makes a really creamy mousse.

Serves 4

Ingredients

135g packet strawberry jelly
Either 125g pot strawberry yoghurt
+ 150ml double cream
    or 125g strawberry soya yoghurt
    + 150ml oat or soya cream
    or 225ml oat cream
6 fresh strawberries

Method

1) Dissolve the jelly in 150ml boiling water and add 150ml cold water. Stir well. Cool in the refrigerator until the jelly is starting to set.

2) Place your choice of yoghurt or cream or cream together with the semi-set jelly in a liquidiser or food processor. Blend together well then pour into 6 ramekin dishes or small bowls or glasses and refrigerate for 2-3 hours.

3) Place a fresh strawberry on top of each mousse before serving.

Marshmallow Fudge

Whether it is to sell at school fêtes or munch at home this fudge is a firm favourite with everyone. Using the microwave ensures that this recipe is also a favourite with the cook as it is much quicker and therefore safer than making traditional fudge on the hob.

Makes 16 pieces

Ingredients

100g icing sugar
50g sultanas
100g white marshmallows
Either 2 tablespoon milk
      or 2 tablespoon oat, rice or soya milk
50g granulated sugar
Either 50g butter or margarine
      or 50g dairy-free **&/or** soya-free margarine

Method

1) Sift the icing sugar into a bowl and mix with the sultanas.

2) In a separate bowl, slowly melt the marshmallows with 1 teaspoon of milk in the microwave on full power for 1 minute. Then leave to cool.

3) Place the remaining milk in a clean bowl, and add the sugar and your choice of butter or margarine. Heat for 1-1½ minutes until the sugar has dissolved in the margarine. Stir well.

4) Ask your adult helper to bring the butter or margarine and sugar mixture to the boil, stirring once every minute. (This will take between 3-5 minutes). Stop once the mixture is brown, bubbling and toffee like. (Don't overheat the mixture or it will burn.) The bowl gets very hot so ask your adult helper to remove the bowl from the microwave using oven gloves.

5) Add the melted marshmallow mixture. Then stir in the icing sugar and sultanas. Mix well. Then pour into a greased 15cm square dish and mark into squares.

6) Place in the fridge until firm.

7) Cut into squares and enjoy.

Rice Crispie Bars

You will have to fight off your non-allergic friends (and their parents) to get a fair share of these gooey party cakes.

Makes 12 pieces

Ingredients

Either 60g butter or margarine
      or 60g dairy-free &/or soya-free margarine
200g white marshmallows
150g rice crispy cereal
1 teaspoon vanilla extract

Method

1) Place the butter or margarine in a saucepan and melt over a low heat. Then gradually add the marshmallows and stir until they are completely melted.

2) (Alternatively place the butter or margarine in a microwaveable glass bowl and melt on full power for 30 seconds. Add the marshmallows, stir well and cook for 1 minute. Stir again until the marshmallows are completely melted.)

3) Remove the mixture from the heat or microwave and stir in the vanilla extract and rice crispy cereal.

4) Pour into a 23cm square dish and place in the refrigerator. Leave to set for an hour.

5) Once cool, cut into approx. 18 bars and serve.

Strawberry Dips

Totally indulgent!

Serves 4-8

Ingredients

400g strawberries (still with stalks on)
100g milk, white or 70% + dairy-free &/or soya-free plain chocolate

Method

1) Wash and dry the strawberries.

2) Break up the chocolate and place in a microwave proof bowl. Melt the chocolate (this could take between 40 –90 seconds depending on your microwave so keep checking after every 20 seconds and do not overheat the chocolate or it will burn.).

3) Hold each strawberry by the stalk and dip into the chocolate. Then place on the serving dish and chill before serving.

Recipe Index

Bibliography

The following have been invaluable sources for the research that has underpinned this book:

(Bingley PJ et al, 2004) Longitudinal studies of parents and children study team. *British Medical Journal.* 328, 322-3; West, J. et al (2003) Seroprevalence, correlates, and characteristics of undetected coeliac disease in England. *Gut;* 52:960–965.)

The Complete Guide to Food Allergy and Intolerance by Professor Jonathan Brostoff and Linda Gamlin published Bloomsbury - revised 1998 Bloomsbury

Nutritional Medicine Dr Stephen Davies and Dr Alan Stewart pub 1987 Pan

The Allergy Connection Barbara Paterson published Thorsons 1986

Hidden Food Allergies Is What You Eat Making You Ill? by Patrick Holford and Dr James Braly published 2005 Piatkus Books Ltd

Food Standards Agency www.food.gov.uk

Department of Health www.doh.gov.uk

World Health Organisation www.who.int

We hope you enjoy reading and using the

Dairy-free &/or
Wheat-free &/or
Soya-free BUT
Always Totally Nut-free
Family Cookbook.

Please visit us online at

www.allergyfamilycookbook.com

CPSIA information can be obtained at www.ICGtesting.com
Printed in the USA
BVOW07s1424041213

338167BV00023B/800/P